500 MCQs in Clinical Medicine

First published 2020

ISBN   9798687032513

Introduction

When you begin to write any book on medicine, you expect the medical world to move on a little bit while you are writing. During the months of working on the book new genetic links will be discovered, new disease risk factors identified and new treatments successfully trialled. The seismic changes in medicine in 2020 brought about by COVID-19 have changed permanently how we see patients, how we manage ourselves during our medical practice, and how medical research is conducted. When I started writing this book masks were worn by a few specialist medical practitioners, now they are worn by all. We have been forced to examine closely our own set-in-stone practices for patient care and adapt them as best as we can to this new world.

One thing that will not change of course is that the medical world needs new doctors, and multiple choice questions will remain a part of the assessment of medical students and doctors in training.

This book uses recently published articles to compile five examination papers, providing best of five multiple choice questions touching every aspect of medicine. COVID-19 questions are included covering areas that are as close to solid fact as can be expected at this early stage since discovery of the disease.

The difficulty level of the questions is high, but the book can be used both for undergraduate and post graduate doctors in training to revise for examinations and practice multiple choice question technique.

Writing these books I am often torn between a relief that I have long finished my own training years, and a memory of the thrill I used to get from studying for examinations and (mostly) passing them. The world of medicine is never short of surprises and challenges as this year has shown. Every doctor gets asked would they do it all over again given these difficulties and challenges, or would they advise their own children to embark on a career in medicine. My answer is always yes.

Dr Nicholas O'Keeffe MBBch BAO MICGP MRCPI MMed Sc (SEM) LFOM

September 2020

Contents

Paper 1

1. FEV 1 and FVC:
   a. Values gradually reduce from age 40
   b. Values do not vary between races
   c. Values are generally higher in women than men
   d. Values are higher in shorter people
   e. FEV1/FVC ratio is independent of height, weight and gender

2. The most common symptom of severe COVID 19 is:
   a. Cough
   b. Fever
   c. Fatigue
   d. Sore throat
   e. Dyspnoea

3. The most common initial cardiovascular manifestation of diabetes is:
   a. Acute myocardial infarction
   b. Heart failure
   c. Sudden cardiac death
   d. Atrial fibrillation
   e. Exertional angina

4. Idiopathic pulmonary fibrosis:
   a. Has a better prognosis than interstitial lung disease secondary to connective tissue disease
   b. Responds well to immunosuppressive therapy
   c. May be inherited as an autosomal dominant genetic condition
   d. High resolution CT scanning has eliminated the need for lung biopsy
   e. Trans-bronchial biopsy is the gold standard for making the diagnosis

5. Glucokinase maturity onset diabetes of the young (GCK-MODY):

a. May present with diabetic ketoacidosis
b. Presents only in children
c. Requires insulin treatment at an early stage
d. Does not respond to oral hypoglycaemics
e. Does not lead to microvascular complications

6. Bicuspid aortic valve:

a. Is more common in women
b. Is an indication for antibiotic prophylaxis before dental procedures
c. Strenuous exercise is contraindicated
d. First degree relatives should be screened
e. Regular surveillance is not required if asymptomatic

7. Anti-phospholipid syndrome (APS):

a. Is associated with an increased risk of venous but not arterial thromboembolism
b. Pulmonary embolism is the most common venous thromboembolic site in APS
c. A diagnosis of APS can be made on clinical grounds
d. Seropositivity for lupus anticoagulant, anti-cardiolipin antibody and anti-β2 glycoprotein I antibody incurs a greater risk of thromboembolism than if only one of these antibodies is positive
e. Venous thromboembolism in APS be treated with direct oral anticoagulant medication (DOACs)

8. Vitamin B12 deficiency:

a. May be associated with macrocytosis and hypersegmented neutrophils on blood film
b. Vitamin B12 is entirely dependent on intrinsic factor for its absorption
c. Pernicious anaemia is the most common cause
d. Neurological manifestations are always preceded by haematological manifestations
e. Requires intramuscular replacement therapy

9. Anti-retroviral treatment should be offered to a HIV positive individual once their CD4+ count drops to:
    a.   500 cells per cubic millimetre
    b.   400 cells per cubic millimetre
    c.   350 cells per cubic millimetre
    d.   200 cells per cubic millimetre
    e.   All HIV positive patients shou d be offered anti-retroviral treatment

10. Hepato-pulmonary syndrome:
    a.   Causes dyspnoea on exertion but not at rest
    b.   Causes dyspnoea at rest which eases on exertion
    c.   Causes dyspnoea and hypoxia on lying flat which eases on sitting upright
    d.   Causes dyspnoea and hypoxia when upright which eases on lying flat
    e.   Causes dyspnoea on standing but not sitting

11. Ablation therapy for atrial fibrillation:
    a.   Reduces mortality compared with medical therapy
    b.   Reduces stroke risk compared with medical therapy
    c.   If the patient is on anti-coagulation for atrial fibrillation prior to ablation therapy, this can be stopped if the procedure successfully converts to sinus rhythm
    d.   Repeat ablation procedures are required in most patients
    e.   There is a 1% risk of cardiac tamponade

12. Duchenne muscular dystrophy:
    a.   Is inherited as an autosomal dominant trait
    b.   Has a less severe course than Becker muscular dystrophy
    c.   Is caused by mutations to the muscle dystrophin gene
    d.   Corticosteroids are not useful in treatment
    e.   If suspected serum LDH shou d be checked

13. Weight loss has a positive predictive value for underlying malignancy of:

    a.   80-90%
    b.   50-60%
    c.   20-30%
    d.   5-10%
    e.   0-3%

14. Peptic ulcer disease:

    a.   NSAID (non-steroidal anti-inflammatory drug) use is associated with 90% of cases of peptic ulcer disease
    b.   NSAID use is more likely to be associated with duodenal than gastric ulcers
    c.   Stool antigen testing for Helicobacter pylori is as reliable as urea breath testing
    d.   Psychologist stress is an established risk factor for peptic ulcer disease
    e.   Consumption of alcohol increases the risk of peptic ulcer disease

15. Chronic spontaneous urticaria:

    a.   Can be treated with anti-IgE monoclonal antibody
    b.   The skin lesions may blister and crust
    c.   May be triggered by pressure on the skin
    d.   May benefit from food avoidance and elimination diets
    e.   H2 receptor antagonists are first line in treatment

16. Telogen effluvium:

    a.   Occurs within one week of a triggering incident
    b.   Causes scarring alopecia
    c.   is associated with positive ds-DNA antibodies
    d.   May occur after pregnancy
    e.   Should be treated with topical steroids

17. Which of the following is <u>not</u> a myeloproliferative neoplasm:
     a.   Acute myeloid leukaemia
     b.   Chronic myeloid leukaemia
     c.   Myelofibrosis
     d.   Polycythaemia vera
     e.   Essential thrombocytosis

18. The most common symptom in patients with hereditary haemorrhagic telangiectasia is:
     a.   Epistaxis
     b.   Haematuria
     c.   Vaginal bleeding
     d.   Rectal bleeding
     e.   Haemoptysis

19. Hutchinson's sign:
     a.   Occurs when herpes zoster rash affects the forehead
     b.   Occurs when herpes zoster rash affects the eye
     c.   Occurs when herpes zoster rash affects the nose
     d.   Occurs when herpes zoster rash affects the ear
     e.   Occurs when herpes zoster rash affects the scalp

20. Malaria:
     a.   Is a viral infection
     b.   Can be transmitted only by the female Aedes mosquito
     c.   Non-mosquito transmission has not been described
     d.   Is preventable by vaccination
     e.   Most malaria deaths occur in sub-Saharan Africa

21. The most common clinical manifestation of alpha-1 antitrypsin deficiency is:
    a.   Emphysema
    b.   Liver cirrhosis in children
    c.   Liver cirrhosis in adults
    d.   c-ANCA positive vasculitis
    e.   Panniculitis

22. Hereditary neuropathy with liability to pressure palsies:
    a.   Is more common in men
    b.   Will not present in childhood
    c.   Neuropathy signs and symptoms recover fully in a period of weeks
    d.   Is associated with diffusely increased tendon reflexes
    e.   Is caused by a deletion on chromosome 17

23. Autonomic dysreflexia:
    a.   Occurs only with spinal injuries affecting C7 vertebra or above
    b.   Is a benign, non-life threatening condition
    c.   The first step in management is to commence anti hypertensive medication
    d.   The lower the level of spinal injury the greater the risk
    e.   The initial presenting symptom is usually a headache

24. Marfan syndrome:
    a.   Is inherited as an autosomal dominant disorder
    b.   There is always a family history
    c.   Occurs in males only
    d.   Is associated with short stature
    e.   Is not associated with reduced life expectancy in untreated affected individuals

25. Langerhans cell histiocytosis:

a. May cause neurodegeneration
b. Responds well to antibiotic treatment
c. Responds well to empirical chemotherapy treatment
d. Is a less severe disease in children
e. The majority of patients recover fully

26. Monoclonal gammopathy of undetermined significance:

a. 5% per year will progress to multiple myeloma
b. Requires an M protein of less than 3g/dl for diagnosis
c. A bone marrow biopsy is required for diagnosis
d. IgG type are most likely to progress to multiple myeloma
e. Should be routinely screened for in those over 50 years of age

27. Erythromelalgia:

a. Is characterised by a triad of burning pain, redness and warmth of the extremities
b. May be inherited as an autosomal recessive condition
c. Pain is exacerbated in cold temperatures
d. Symptoms tend to be static over time
e. Symptoms respond well to sodium channel blockers

28. The leading cause of arthropod-borne viral disease in the world is:

a. Yellow fever
b. Dengue fever
c. West Nile virus
d. Chikungunya
e. Zika virus

29. The 'nocebo' effect:

a. Refers to the induction or worsening of adverse symptoms while taking a sham or active treatment
b. Refers to the reduction of adverse effects of a medication while taking a sham or active treatment
c. Refers to a perceived benefit in an individual taking a sham or active treatment
d. Refers to increased mortality occurring in a group taking a sham or active treatment
e. Refers to a reduction in mortality occurring in a group taking a sham or active treatment

30. Legionnaire's disease:

a. Has a mortality of 60% when community-acquired
b. Can be diagnosed reliably with a urinary antigen test
c. Early antibiotic treatment does not affect mortality
d. Diarrhoea is not a frequent symptom
e. All cases are caused by Legionella pneumophila

31. Cystic fibrosis:

a. Siblings of an affected individual have a 75% chance of being affected
b. Occurs due to excess water in mucoid secretions
c. 99% of affected males are infertile
d. Sweat testing is insensitive and non-specific
e. A minority will have pancreatic insufficiency

32. Hypertrophic cardiomyopathy (HCM):

a. Requires asymmetric septal hypertrophy for diagnosis
b. Affected individuals have an increased risk of atrial fibrillation
c. Is the leading cause of sudden cardiac death in athletes
d. Affected individuals should avoid golf
e. ACE inhibitors are useful for reducing left ventricular outflow obstruction

33. The most useful investigation in diagnosing ankylosing spondylitis is:
    a. HLA 27 testing
    b. Inflammatory markers ESR and CRP
    c. X ray sacroiliac joints
    d. MRI sacroiliac joints
    e. MRI lumbosacral spine

34. Prolactin:
    a. Is most active in its polymeric macroprolactin form
    b. Dopamine stimulates prolactin release
    c. Oestrogens enhance prolactin release
    d. Breast ultrasound and mammography may induce hyperprolactinaemia
    e. Should be measured in early morning

35. Sickle cell disease:
    a. Compound heterozygotes for the HbS gene and other haemoglobin abnormalities usually have more severe clinical manifestations that those with sickle cell disease
    b. Those with sickle cell disease and α-thalassaemia have more severe haemolysis than those with sickle-cell disease alone
    c. Those with sickle cell disease and α-thalassaemia have more severe vaso-occlusive sickle cell complications
    d. Higher HbF levels in those with sickle cell are associated with more severe disease
    e. Those with sickle cell disease will not contract malaria

36. The intervention with the greatest impact on the natural history of chronic obstructive pulmonary disease is:
    a. Smoking cessation
    b. Inhaled long acting beta-agonist
    c. Inhaled long acting muscarinic antagonists
    d. Pulmonary rehabilitation
    e. Influenza vaccination

37. Tuberculosis and BCG vaccination:
    a.   BCG vaccine should always be given intramuscularly
    b.   Evidence of the protective effects of BCG is stronger in adults than young children
    c.   BCG should not be given within three months of another live vaccine
    d.   BCG vaccination should be given to those with HIV
    e.   There is no proven benefit in giving BCG over the age of 35 years of age

38. IgA nephropathy:
    a.   Most commonly presents with acute kidney injury
    b.   Peak incidence is in in the 7th decade
    c.   ACE-inhibitors are contraindicated
    d.   Definitive diagnosis requires kidney biopsy
    e.   Rarely progresses to end-stage renal disease

39. Sarcoidosis:
    a.   Has a well-understood aetiology
    b.   Has its highest incidence in those of Asian origin
    c.   The organ most commonly affected is the skin
    d.   The presence of non-caseating granulomas on biopsy is sufficient for diagnosis
    e.   Methotrexate is the first-line steroid-sparing agent in treatment

40. Dermatomyositis:
    a.   Autoantibodies are usually negative
    b.   Affected individuals should be evaluated for possible malignancy
    c.   Muscle biopsy finding are histopathologically indistinguishable from polymyositis
    d.   Asymmetrical proximal muscle weakness is a hallmark clinical feature
    e.   Heliotrope rash may occur on the hands

41. Troponins:
- a. Are sensitive but not specific markers for myocardial damage
- b. Have a high negative predictive value in ruling out a cardiac cause for chest pain
- c. Troponin I, troponin C and troponin T are specific for myocardium
- d. Are useful in diagnosis but not prognosis in acute coronary syndrome
- e. Do not have a diurnal variation

42. Syphilis:
- a. Is a parasitic infection
- b. May be spread to humans from animals
- c. Non-sexual spread has not been described
- d. Presents with a painless genital chancre in its primary stage
- e. Primary syphilis is not infectious

43. Insulinoma:
- a. May present with seizures
- b. Normal insulin levels exclude insulinoma
- c. Is usually malignant
- d. First-line treatment is non-surgical
- e. May occur in MEN II syndrome

44. A lung nodule is defined as:
- a. A well-defined rounded opacity measuring up to 5cm in diameter
- b. A well-defined rounded opacity measuring up to 4cm in diameter
- c. A well-defined rounded opacity measuring up to 3cm in diameter
- d. A well-defined rounded opacity measuring up to 2cm in diameter
- e. A well-defined rounded opacity measuring up to 1cm in diameter

45. The most common valvular heart disease is:
    a. Aortic stenosis
    b. Aortic regurgitation
    c. Mitral stenosis
    d. Mitral regurgitation
    e. Tricuspid regurgitation

46. The 2009 'swine flu' pandemic was caused by:
    a. Influenza A (H5N1)
    b. Influenza A (H1N1)
    c. Influenza A (H3N2)
    d. Influenza A (H2N2)
    e. Influenza A (H3N8)

47. ANCA-associated vasculitis:
    a. Primarily affects large blood vessels
    b. Microscopic polyangiitis was formerly known as Wegener's granulomatosis
    c. May be a cause of sensorineural deafness
    d. Renal involvement is the most common manifestation
    e. Life expectancy is similar to that of the general population with treatment

48. Bowen's disease:
    a. Lesions are usually itchy
    b. Lesions are usually ulcerated
    c. High risk lesions are on the ear, nose, lip, or eyelid or have a diameter of over 10 mm
    d. Rarely progresses to squamous cell carcinoma
    e. Increases quickly in size over weeks to months

49. Acute respiratory distress syndrome:
a. Will only occur secondary to pulmonary infection
b. Mortality rate is 5-10%
c. Usually responds well to antibiotics
d. Steroids have been shown to reduce mortality
e. Can be classified into mild, moderate and severe depending on level of hypoxaemia

50. Fanconi anaemia:
a. Is the same as Fanconi syndrome
b. Is characterised by tall stature
c. Red blood cells are the only blood line affected
d. There is an increased risk of leukaemia but not an increased risk of solid tumours
e. Androgens may be used in treatment

51. Benign liver lesions:
a. Are associated with exogenous oestrogen use
b. Hepatic adenomas are the most common
c. They are more common in men
d. Generally require surveillance
e. Will not undergo malignant transformation

52. Neurocysticercosis:
a. Only humans and cows act as hosts of the causative agent
b. Disease affecting the brain parenchyma has a worse prognosis than extra parenchymal disease
c. May present with hydrocephalus
d. Most commonly presents with facial palsy
e. Should be treated immediately with anti-parasitic medication

53. Multiple sclerosis:
a. Clinically isolated syndrome lasts at least 24 hours
b. Progressive type is more common than relapsing-remitting type
c. Treatment does not prevent relapse and future disability
d. Can be diagnosed on the basis of an initial presentation of bilateral optic neuritis
e. Can be diagnosed based on MRI scan findings only

54. Nikolsky sign occurs in:
a. Eczema
b. Psoriasis
c. Stevens-Johnson syndrome
d. Bullous pemphigoid
e. Spontaneous urticaria

55. Which of the following corticosteroids will have the most anti-inflammatory potency per mg dose:
a. Cortisone
b. Prednisolone
c. Fludrocortisone
d. Dexamethasone
e. Triamcinolone

56. Severe acute respiratory syndrome (SARS):
a. Is an interchangeable term with adult respiratory distress syndrome (ARDS)
b. Is an infectious condition transmitted primarily via the respiratory route
c. Rhinorrhoea is a frequent presenting symptom
d. Lymphocytosis is a common feature
e. Has a higher mortality rate in children than in the elderly

57. Cephalosporins:
  a. Should not be given to those with a history of penicillin allergy
  b. Share a similar molecular structure to penicillin
  c. Allergy to one cephalosporin implies allergy to all cephalosporins
  d. Have a narrow spectrum of antibacterial action
  e. IgE mediated cephalosporin allergy is common

58. Drug reaction with eosinophilia and systemic symptoms (DRESS syndrome):
  a. Myocarditis may occur up to 4 months after initial presentation
  b. May present with autoimmune disease up to three years later the most common of which is Addison's disease
  c. Skin rash typically presents within 24 hours of drug exposure
  d. Does not occur in children
  e. Can be excluded if the rash is not morbilliform

59. Methotrexate:
  a. Oral methotrexate has been shown to have greater efficacy and tolerability than subcutaneously administered methotrexate
  b. Is primarily excreted by the liver
  c. Is a folate antagonist
  d. Folic acid supplementation may reduce the anti-inflammatory effect of methotrexate in rheumatological disease
  e. Can be given in a daily dosage

60. Primary ciliary dyskinesia (PCD):
  a. Normal ciliary ultrastructure on biopsy excludes the diagnosis
  b. Is always associated with organ laterality defects such as situs inversus
  c. Nasal saccharine clearance test is useful in diagnosis
  d. Nasal nitric oxide tends to be higher in those with PCD
  e. Bronchiectasis is present in all adults in PCD

61. Which of the following is <u>not</u> a component of the CHA2DS2-VASc score for stroke risk stratification in atrial fibrillation:
    a.   Age
    b.   Congestive cardiac failure
    c.   Valvular heart disease
    d.   Diabetes mellitus
    e.   Previous stoke/TIA

62. Cutaneous T cell lymphoma:
    a.   Involves infiltration of the skin by monoclonal malignant T cells
    b.   The most common is Sezary syndrome
    c.   Is curable
    d.   LDH levels are specific in diagnosis
    e.   Topical treatments are not useful

63. Which of the following is not a typical clinical feature of Parkinson's disease:
    a.   Asymmetrical rest tremor
    b.   Bradykinesia
    c.   Motor weakness
    d.   Postural instability
    e.   Rigidity

64. Which of the following conditions is <u>not</u> associated with an increased risk of coeliac disease:
    a.   Down's syndrome
    b.   Grave's disease
    c.   Type 2 diabetes
    d.   IgA deficiency
    e.   Psoriasis

65. Lipomas:

a.   Should always be removed
b.   Are usually fixed to the underlying tissue
c.   Are more common in diabetes
d.   Are most commonly greater than 10cm diameter
e.   Are usually painful

66. Non-alcoholic fatty liver disease (NAFLD):

a.   Requires liver biopsy for diagnosis and management
b.   Will not progress to liver cirrhosis
c.   Fibrosis can be accurately detected on liver ultrasound
d.   May occur in up to 90% of those with diabetes mellitus
e.   Will not occur in those with a normal BMI (18.5-24.9)

67. Non-secreting pituitary adenomas:

a.   Typically present with signs of raised gonadotropin levels such as ovarian hyperstimulation and increased testicular size
b.   Rarely recur after surgical resection
c.   Visual defect is typically a homonymous hemianopia
d.   Visual deficits are not restored after surgical resection
e.   10% present with pituitary apoplexy

68. Rinne test:

a.   Should be performed using a 256Hz tuning fork
b.   Is negative when air conduction s greater than bone conduction
c.   May be a false negative if there is a profound conductive hearing loss in the tested ear
d.   May be a false negative if there is a profound sensorineural hearing loss in the tested ear
e.   True Rinne negative requires a hearing loss of at least 40 decibels

69. Phocomelia is:

a. An acquired brain injury from trauma
b. Limb deformities arising from thalidomide exposure
c. Visual disturbance arising from hydroxychloroquine exposure
d. Hearing impairment arising from aminoglycoside exposure
e. Proximal myopathy arising from long term exogenous corticosteroid exposure

70. Q fever:

a. Is caused by Francisella tularensis
b. Antibiotic treatment is not needed
c. Inhalation is the most common route of transmission
d. Is caused by a spore-forming organism
e. Is transmitted to humans only from goats

71. Chronic atrophic gastritis:

a. Increases the risk of stomach malignancy
b. Will present with macrocytic but not microcytic anaemia
c. Risk is not increased with the presence of helicobacter pylori infection
d. Is increased in those with type 2 diabetes
e. Causes excessive acid secretion in the stomach

72. If a substance is classified as a group 2a carcinogen by the International Agency for Research on Cancer this indicates that the substance:

a. Is not carcinogenic to humans
b. Is not classifiable as regards its carcinogenicity
c. Is possibly carcinogenic to humans
d. Is probably carcinogenic to humans
e. Is known to be carcinogenic to humans

73. Which of the following is <u>not</u> associated with an increased risk of hidradenitis suppurativa:
    a.   Smoking
    b.   Obesity
    c.   Spondyloarthropathy
    d.   Positive family history
    e.   Low body mass index (<18)

74. Oseltamivir:
    a.   Reduces hospitalisation rates from influenza
    b.   Reduces rates of pneumonia following influenza
    c.   Reduces rates of death from influenza
    d.   Reduces duration of symptoms from influenza by on average less than 24 hours
    e.   Is taken via inhalation

75. Primary hyperparathyroidism:
    a.   The distal third of the radius is particular sensitive to cortical loss in primary hyperparathyroidism
    b.   10% occurs due to parathyroid carcinoma
    c.   80% occurs due to hyperplasia of all four parathyroid glands
    d.   Increases the risk of hip fracture
    e.   May occur due to inflammatory bowel disease

76. Long-term macrolide use in asthma:
    a.   Is not currently recommended
    b.   Improves FEV1
    c.   Reduces exacerbations
    d.   Reduces inhaled corticosteroid use
    e.   Reduces hospitalisation risk

77. The most common sustained arrhythmia is:

    a.   First degree heart block
    b.   Atrial fibrillation
    c.   Atrial flutter
    d.   Junctional tachycardia
    e.   Complete heart block

78. SARS CoV-2:

    a.   Is a DNA virus
    b.   Enters human cells through the angiotensin converter enzyme-1 (ACE-1) receptor
    c.   Is spread only via aerosol
    d.   Is usually diagnosed via serology
    e.   Causes mild illness in approximately 80% of those infected

79. Bechet's disease:

    a.   Vasculitis can affect both veins and arteries
    b.   Occurs most commonly over the age of 65
    c.   Oral ulcers are usually painless
    d.   Ocular involvement is rare
    e.   Venous thrombosis occurs in 90% of cases

80. Lipids:

    a.   A statin should only be started in those with diabetes if the 10 year risk of cardiovascular disease is >20%
    b.   Statins inhibit f 3-hydroxy-3-methylglutaryl coenzyme A (HMG-CoA) reductase which leads to reduced expression of the hepatic LDL receptor and reduced clearance of LDL from the circulation
    c.   Statins reduce the risk of developing diabetes mellitus
    d.   The benefits of statin therapy are greatest in its first year
    e.   Ezetimibe has not been shown to improve cardiovascular outcomes when used in isolation

81. Haemochromatosis:

- a. The most common genetic mutation in haemochromatosis is a G-to-A missense mutation leading to the substitution of tyrosine for cysteine at amino acid position 282 of the protein product
- b. Homozygosity for a relevant gene is sufficient for diagnosis
- c. Transferrin saturation reflects the amount of serum iron stored as ferritin
- d. First degree relatives of an affected individual should be screened with iron study testing but not with genetic testing
- e. Venesection of 500ms of blood removes 500mg of iron

82. Hodgkin's lymphoma:

- a. Nodular lymphocyte predominant has a more aggressive course then classical Hodgkin's lymphoma
- b. Lymphocyte depleted classical Hodgkin's lymphoma is the rarest subtype of classical Hodgkin's lymphoma and has the most aggressive course
- c. Mixed cellularity type is the most common type of classical Hodgkin's lymphoma
- d. Nodular sclerosis has the worse prognosis of the classical Hodgkin's lymphoma subtypes
- e. Lymphocyte rich classical lymphoma tends to present with bulky mediastinal adenopathy

83. Which of the following has not been associated with increased risk of Crohn's disease:

- a. Antibiotic use
- b. Vaccines
- c. Regular use of non-steroidal anti-inflammatory drugs
- d. Smoking
- e. Homozygosity for NOD 2 gene

84. Propranolol:

- a. Reduces exogenous thyroxine levels
- b. Reduces circulating serum T_3 levels
- c. Reduces circulating endogenous serum T_4 levels
- d. Reduces circulating serum TSH levels
- e. Has no effect on thyroid hormone levels

85. Obstructive sleep apnoea:

a. An apnoea-hypopnoea index of >5 indicates severe obstructive sleep apnoea

b. Use of continuous positive airway pressure (CPAP) for 4 hours per night for 50% of the time is considered good adherence to treatment

c. It is known to increase the risk of road traffic accidents by 10%

d. Severe obstructive sleep apnoea has been shown to increase all-cause and cardiovascular mortality

e. Does not occur in those with a non-obese body mass index

86. D Dimer testing:

a. Is most useful where the pre-test probability of venous thromboembolic disease is high

b. Levels gradually reduce in pregnancy between the first and third trimesters

c. Levels increase with advancing age

d. Is not useful for predicting recurrence of venous thromboembolic disease

e. An elevated D Dimer level is sufficient to diagnose disseminated intravascular coagulation (DIC)

87. Which of the following is required for a diagnosis of Harlequin syndrome:

a. Anisocoria

b. Unilateral ptosis

c. Excessive flushing and sweating on one side of the face with exertion

d. Permanent facial discoloration

e. Unilateral flushing and sweating affecting the whole body

88. Ebola virus disease is caused by a:

a. Parvovirus

b. Filovirus

c. Coronavirus

d. Orthomyxovirus

e. Adenovirus

89. Heart failure with preserved ejection fraction (HFpEF):
     a.   Is often asymptomatic
     b.   Will have normal brain-natriuretic peptide levels
     c.   Is characterised by an ejection fraction of >50%
     d.   Loop diuretics will not improve symptoms in HFpEF
     e.   ACE inhibitors reduce mortality in HFpEF

90. Necrotising fasciitis:
     a.   Is rarely fatal
     b.   Most commonly affects post operative wounds
     c.   Is best diagnosed by skin biopsy
     d.   Plain film radiology is the best radiological modality to
          aid diagnosis
     e.   Requires prompt surgical treatment

91. Which of the following do <u>not</u> increase risk of developing ulcerative colitis:
     a.   Family history of ulcerative colitis
     b.   Former cigarette smoking
     c.   History of acute appendicitis
     d.   Urban living
     e.   Non-steroidal anti-inflammatory drug use

92. Infective endocarditis:
     a.   The most common risk factor in the developed world
          is rheumatic heart disease
     b.   There is 100% mortality if untreated
     c.   Enterococci are the most common pathogen
     d.   Blood cultures are negative in 50% of cases
     e.   Occurs more commonly in a structurally normal than a
          structurally abnormal heart

93. Medications used in type 2 diabetes that improve glycaemic control by reducing glucose reabsorption in the renal proximal tubule are known as:
   a. Dipeptyl peptidase-4 (DPP-4) inhibitors
   b. Glucagon-like peptide 1 (GLP-1) agonists
   c. Sulphonylureas
   d. Thiazolidinediones
   e. Sodium-glucose cotransporter 2 (SGLT-2) inhibitors

94. α - thalassaemia:
   a. There are over 100 known genetic forms
   b. α chains come from a single gene locus
   c. Defective production of α chains lead to excess γ chains in an adult
   d. Is not protective against malaria
   e. The $α^+$-thalassaemia is more severe than the $α^0$-thalassaemia form

95. Graft vs host disease (GVHD):
   a. Occurs when donor B cells recognise the host as foreign
   b. Jaundice is the most common presenting feature of acute GVHD
   c. A female donor and a male recipient increases risk
   d. Can occur due to disparities with minor histocompatibility antigen (miH) but not major histocompatibility complexes (MHC) between donor and host
   e. Corticosteroids are not useful in treatment

96. Nutcracker syndrome:
   a. Occurs due to compression of the right renal vein between the aorta and the superior mesenteric artery
   b. Occurs only in men
   c. Prevalence peaks over the age of 70
   d. May cause visible haematuria
   e. Does not require surgical intervention

97. Which of the following is the most useful investigation in the acute settling in an individual diagnosed with a recent transient ischaemic attack:
    a. ECG
    b. CRP
    c. CT scan of brain
    d. Diffusion weighted imaging assessed with MRI scan
    e. MR angiography

98. The sensitivity of a test refers to:
    a. The proportion of people with a condition who have a positive test result
    b. The proportion of people without a condition who have a negative test result
    c. The proportion of people with a condition who have a negative test result
    d. The proportion of people without a condition who have a positive test result
    e. The proportion of people with a condition with a given test result (either positive or negative) divided by the proportion of people without the condition with that result

99. Tumour lysis syndrome:
    a. Spontaneous TLS is more common than chemotherapy induced TLS
    b. Laboratory tumour lysis syndrome does not require treatment
    c. Hypercalcaemia is the earliest biochemical manifestation
    d. Acute kidney injury is the most common clinical manifestation
    e. Is most commonly associated with lung cancer

100. Tetanus:
    a. Localised tetanus is more common than generalised tetanus
    b. Most cases develop within 14 days of exposure
    c. The longer the incubation period the greater the risk of death
    d. Cannot be treated with antibiotics
    e. Is diagnosed by culture of the organism

1. Answer e

FEV1 (forced expiratory volume in 1 second) and FVC (forced vital capacity) gradually reduce from about age 20. Individual values are higher in men. Black Africans have 10-15% lower values than Caucasians for a given height. Although the interpretation of FEV1 and FVC readings is dependent on height, weight and gender, the FEV1/FVC ratio self-normalises.[30]

2. Answer e

The most common symptom of severe COVID 19 is dyspnoea which may be accompanied by severe hypoxaemia. Severe Covid-19 in adults is characterised by dyspnoea, a respiratory rate of 30 or more breaths per minute, a blood oxygen saturation of 93% or less, a ratio of the partial pressure of arterial oxygen to the fraction of inspired oxygen ($PaO_2:FIO_2$) of less than 300 mm Hg, or infiltrates on x ray of more than 50% of the lung field within 24 to 48 hours from the onset of symptoms.[149]

3. Answer b

Heart failure is the most common initial cardiovascular manifestation of diabetes and a more common reason for emergency admission in patients with diabetes than acute myocardial infarction or stroke.[2] Diabetic cardiomyopathy is considered a distinct pathological entity with signs of cardiac dysfunction without evidence of coronary artery disease, hypertension or congenital or valvular heart disease. Metabolic abnormalities associated with diabetes are believed to have an effect on myocardium leading to heart failure.

4. Answer c

Idiopathic pulmonary fibrosis has a poor prognosis, often worse than some lung cancers. It responds poorly to immunosuppressive therapy and tends to have a worse prognosis than interstitial lung disease from secondary causes. Some cases are familial and can be inherited in an autosomal dominant manner. High resolution CT scanning has revolutionised the diagnosis of interstitial lung disease but lung biopsy is still needed in some cases. Transbronchial biopsy does not always obtain sufficient tissue for diagnosis and surgical biopsy is the gold standard for diagnosis but is usually not necessary.[3]

5. Answer e

1-2% of diabetes is a monogenic type known as maturity onset diabetes of the young (MODY). It is a distinct entity from type 1 and type 2 diabetes. The most common types involve genes encoding the enzyme glucokinase (GCK) and the nuclear transcription factors hepatocyte nuclear factor 1α (HNF1A) and hepatocyte nuclear factor 4α (HNF4A). GCK-MODY results in stable long-term hyperglycaemia with no treatment needed with insulin or hypoglycaemics. It may show up incidentally on routine blood testing at any age. It does not lead to microvascular complications.

HNF1A- MODY and HNF4A-MODY lead to progressively worsening hyperglycaemia into adulthood and can lead to microvascular complications. They are not associated with insulin resistance but do not respond to insulin. Patients with these conditions are very sensitive to sulphonylurea medication which is usually the treatment of choice.[4]

6. Answer d

Bicuspid aortic valve is one of the most common congenital cardiac abnormalities and can lead to aortic valve and aortic root abnormalities as well as thoracic aortic aneurysm and dissection. There is also an increased risk of endocarditis. It is more common in men. Antibotic prophylaxis is not needed before dental procedures in the absence of previous endocarditis. Strenuous exercise is only a risk if there is associated dilatation of the ascending aorta. Those with bicuspid aortic valve and normal ascending aorta have no exercise restrictions. There can be a familial element and first -degree relatives should be screened. Regular surveillance with transthoracic echocardiogram is required, usually every 5 to 10 years in those with no signs of aortic valve or ascending aorta abnormalities.[5]

7. Answer d

Anti-phospholipid syndrome (APS) is diagnosed based on a history of venous or arterial thromboembolism and/or or a history of specifically defined obstetric complications in combination with seropositivity for one of the anti-phospholipid antibodies (lupus anticoagulant, anti-cardiolipin antibody and anti-β2 glycoprotein I antibody). The deep veins of the leg are the most common site for venous thromboembolism in APS. Triple seropositivity incurs the greatest risk for recurrent thrombosis. The safety and efficacy of direct oral anticoagulants have not been established in APS and warfarin should be used to treat venous thromboembolism.[8]

8. Answer a

Pernicious anaemia is responsible for a minority of cases of vitamin B12 deficiency, with food-bound cobalamin malabsorption (FBCM) the most common cause now. A small proportion (1-5%) of vitamin B12 is absorbed in an intrinsic-factor independent diffusion process. Neurological manifestations may present without haematological abnormalities, and vice versa. There is increasing evidence that oral replacement is sufficient in most cases of vitamin B12 deficiency.[9]

9. Answer e

The Strategic Timing of Antiretroviral Therapy (START) trial published in 2015 showed benefit in patients started on anti-retroviral therapy at an early stage, with CD4+ counts higher than 500 cells per cubic millimetre. Benefits were seen in serious AIDS-related and serious non-AIDS related outcomes after three years without significant adverse effects to outweigh the benefits. All patients with HIV should be offered anti-retroviral treatment.[10]

10. Answer d

Hepato-pulmonary syndrome may occur in decompensated liver disease and is characterised by a triad of liver dysfunction, intrapulmonary vasodilatation and arterial oxygenation defect. It leads to platypnoea and orthodeoxia (dyspnoea and hypoxia worse in the upright position and improved on lying flat.[11]

11. Answer e

Ablation therapy for atrial fibrillation involves using radiofrequency ablation or cryoablation to destroy foci of aberrant electrical activity at the junction between the pulmonary veins and left atrium. It has not been shown to reduce stroke risk or mortality but may improve quality of life. It may also be more beneficial than medical therapy in those who have atrial fibrillation and heart failure. It is recommended in those with symptomatic atrial fibrillation who have not responded to or wish to avoid anti-arrhythmic medications. Anti-coagulation should be continued post-ablation (if indicated by $CHA_2 DS_2$ -VASC risk score) even if the procedure is successful as this population are shown to have increased risk of stroke compared to those with no history of atrial fibrillation. Repeat ablation procedures are required in 20-40% of cases. Cardiac tamponade, stroke, pulmonary vein stenosis and atrio-oesophageal fistula are among the risks.[12]

12. Answer c

Duchenne muscular dystrophy is a condition characterised by muscle degeneration caused by mutations to the muscle dystrophin gene. It is inherited in an X-linked recessive manner so it mostly affects boys. Becker muscular dystrophy is also caused by mutations to muscle dystrophin genes but presents later with an overall slower progression. Corticosteroid treatment has been shown to slow progression of muscle deterioration in Duchenne muscular dystrophy and patients may survive into their thirties with treatment. If the condition is suspected then creatinine kinase (CK) should be checked urgently as this is always raised.[13]

13. Answer e

A history of weight loss has a positive predictive value of 0-3% for underlying malignancy.[14]

14. Answer c

NSAID use is associated with 10% of peptic ulcer disease and is more associated with gastric than duodenal ulcers. Stool antigen testing is as reliable as urea breath testing for Helicobacter pylori. Neither psychological stress nor alcohol use are proven risk factors for peptic ulcer disease.[15]

15. Answer a

Chronic spontaneous urticaria is urticarial rash without a trigger lasting at least 6 weeks continuously or intermittently. First line treatment is with second generation non-sedating H1 receptor antihistamines. H2 receptor antihistamines such as ranitidine are not thought to be helpful. The anti-IgE monoclonal antibody omalizumab can be used in treatment. Urticarial rash does not blister or scar, this would be more consistent with erythema multiforme, a differential diagnosis. Urticaria may be caused by external stimulants such as pressure but this is known as inducible urticaria, a separate condition. Food avoidance and dietary elimination are not helpful in chronic spontaneous urticaria.[16]

16. Answer d

Telogen effluvium involves non-scarring hair loss occurring 2 to 3 months after a triggering event such as psychological stress, febrile illness or pregnancy. It occurs due to disruption of the usual anagen (growing hair), catagen (involuting hair) and telogen (resting hair) cycle that may lead to simultaneous loss of multiple hair follicles. It is usually self-limiting and spontaneous hair regrowth usually occurs, but may take 12 to 18 months. It may in some cases progress to chronic telogen effluvium. There is no diagnostic blood test. There is no specific treatment unless there is an associated deficiency.[17]

17. Answer a

The myeloproliferative neoplasms are essential thrombocytosis, chronic myeloid leukaemia, polycythaemia vera and myelofibrosis. The WHO classification of myeloproliferative neoplasms also includes chronic neutrophilic leukaemia, chronic eosinophilic leukaemia and MPN unclassifiable. Myeloproliferative neoplasms are characterised by monoclonal proliferation of myeloid cells in the peripheral blood and bone marrow, and the cells retain the ability to differentiate to red blood cells, white blood cells or platelets. They may overlap and are linked by a group of driver genetic mutations (JAK2, CALR and MPL). They may have similar clinical and lab characteristics such as splenomegaly and raised red blood cells and/or white blood cells and/or platelets. Myeloproliferative neoplasms may transform to acute myeloid leukaemia which has a poor prognosis.[18]

18. Answer a

Hereditary haemorrhagic telangiectasia is a condition characterised by cutaneous, mucosal and visceral telangiectasia and visceral arteriovenous malformations. It is caused by three genetic mutaticns leading to abnormal blood vessel development. The most common symptom is epistaxis.[19]

19. Answer c

Hutchinson's sign refers to rash affecting the nose in herpes zoster ophthalmicus and is an indicator of likely corneal involvement due to the common nerve supply through the nasociliary branch of the trigeminal nerve.[20]

20. Answer e

Malaria is a parasitic infection caused by the Plasmodium species, transmitted by the female Anopheles mosquito. Transmission without a mosquito is rare but may occur via vertical transmission from mother to child congenitally, via organ transplantation, blood transfusion or needle sharing. There is no known vaccination. 90% of deaths occur in sub-Saharan Africa.[21,22,23]

21. Answer a

All of the above are associated with alpha-1 antitrypsin deficiency but emphysema is the most common clinical manifestation.[24]

22. Answer e

Hereditary neuropathy with liability to pressure palsies is an autosomal dominant condition with predisposition to symptomat c peripheral pressure palsies such as carpal tunnel syndrome or foot drop. It usually presents with mononeuropathies, most commonly affecting the median nerve, ulnar nerve, peroneal nerve at the fibular head causing foor drop, and the brachial plexus and radial nerve causing sensory hand symptoms. Full recovery occurs in 50% of episodes so disability can persist. It most commonly presents in the second and third decades but first presentation has been described from age 2 to 70. Men and women are equally affected. It is associated with reduced generalised tendon reflexes. It is caused by a deletion at chromosome 17p11.2 affecting the PMP22 gene.[25]

23. Answer e

Autonomic dysreflexia occurs in those who have suffered a severe spinal injury. It occurs due to autonomic dysregulation causing an uncoordinated autonomic response leading to severe hypertension due to a stimulus below the level of the spinal injury. It occurs in spinal injuries above the level of T6, and the higher the level of spinal injury the greater the risk. It is a potentially life threatening condition and may cause haemorrhagic stroke. It may occur due to triggers such as bladder or rectal distension, but there are other potential stimuli. The first step in management is to look for a trigger and manage this, but antihypertensive medication may be needed. It initially presents with headache.[26]

24. Answer a

Marfan syndrome is an autosomal dominant disorder characterised by mutations to the fibrillin 1 (FBN1) gene, affecting the pliability of connective tissues. It can affect many organ systems and varies in its clinical severity. 25% are sporadic mutations without a family history. There is no preference for gender. It is associated with tall stature. Life expectancy is considerably shortened to about 32 years due to aortic root complications although treatments now are improving this.[27,28]

25. Answer a

Langerhans cell histiocytosis was formerly called histiocytosis. Further understanding of its pathogenesis has emerged in recent years and it is now understood to arise due to misguided myeloid differentiation leading to granulomatous lesions of epidermal dendritic (Langerhans) cells and inflammatory infiltrate. It varies hugely in its severity from isolated indolent lesions to rapid progressive illness in children. Antibiotics are not used in treatment, and the usual treatment of vincristine and prednisolone fails to cure over half of patients. 5% will suffer a neurodegenerative condition and most patients are left with long term sequelae.[29]

26. Answer b

Monoclonal gammopathy of undetermired significance (MGUS) is a monoclonal proliferation of plasma cells leading to excess protein on serum protein electrophoresis known as an M protein. 1% per year or less progress to myeloma. The IgM type is the most likely to progress. MGUS requires an M protein level of less than 3g/dl on serum protein electrophoresis and less than 10% clonal cells in the bone marrow in the absence of myeloma-related end-organ damage. A bone marrow biopsy is not required in low-risk MGUS. MGUS tends to be detected during investigations for conditions such as anaemia or neuropathy and should not be screened for routinely.[31]

27. Answer a

Erythromelalgia is a painful condition characterised by a triad of burning pain, redness and warmth of the extremities, often triggered by warm environments or exercise. Primary erythromelalgia is an autosomal dominant condition occurring due to mutation at SCN9A, a gene encoding a voltage-gated sodium channel. Erythromelalgia may be secondary to conditions such as myeloproliferative disorder or secondary to certain medications such as calcium channel blockers. It is a debilitating condition refractory to most treatments and with progression in most people over time. It may lead to gangrene and ulceration of the extremities due to repeated self-exposure to cold in an attempt to relieve symptoms.[32]

28. Answer b

Dengue fever is the fastest-spreading mosquito-borne viral disease, now infecting more than 100 million people annually and causing up to 25000 deaths.[33]

29. Answer a

'Nocebo' effect refers to the induction or worsening of symptoms in individuals taking a sham or active treatment. It is the negative version of the placebo effect. An example would be statin associated muscle symptoms, which have been shown to be induced by placebo in some trials.[37,38]

30. Answer b

Legionnaire's disease is caused by Legionella bacteria, most commonly Legionella pneumophila. It is probably under-diagnosed but can have a severe course with a mortality rate of up to 20% in susceptible individuals. There is increased susceptibility in men, in those aged over 50 years, and in smokers and in those with chronic lung disease. It can be diagnosed with a urinary antigen test and early treatment with macrolide antibiotics alters the course of the illness. 90% of Legionnaire's disease is caused by Legionella pneumophila with the remainder caused by other Legionella serotypes.[39]

31. Answer c

Cystic fibrosis is a disorder of chloride transport in exocrine glands resulting from mutations to the cystic fibrosis transmembrane conductance regulator (CFTR) gene on chromosome 7. It is inherited in an autosomal recessive pattern and so siblings of affected individuals have a 25% chance of being affected. Reduced chloride secretion leads to increased sodium and water uptake and viscous mucoid secretions. Testing for chloride measurement in sweat is 96.5% sensitive and 99% specific if performed properly. 99% of affected males are infertile due to obstructive azoospermia and 87% of affected individuals will have pancreatic insufficiency.[40]

32. Answer b

Hypertrophic cardiomyopathy (HCM) is a genetic condition of the myocardium, which is inherited in an autosomal dominant manner or may be sporadic. Asymmetric septal hypertrophy is characteristic but not always present and left ventricular hypertrophy may be concentric or may affect other walls or the apex. Diagnosis is made based on ventricular wall thickness of >15mm at its maximum, or >13mm in the presence of a family history or positive genetic testing. There is an increased risk of atrial fibrillation among other arrhythmias. It was historically thought to be the most common cause of sudden cardiac death in athletes but more recent studies have cast doubt on this. Most affected individuals are restricted from vigorous exercise, although less rigorous sports such as bowls and golf are not necessarily contraindicated. More recently a more liberal stance has been taken with regard to exercise in HCM, and also with an increased understanding of the risks of a sedentary lifestyle in those with HCM, some exercise is encouraged in low risk individuals. Caution and expert advice is needed for such recommendations. Medical management such as beta blockers can be used to reduced outflow tract gradient and for their negative chronotropic effect to improve diastolic filing, but ACE inhibitors and diuretics may be harmful.[41,42,43,44]

33. Answer d

Axial spondyloarthropathies are divided into spondyloarthropathy with radiographic changes in the sacro-iliac joints (radiographic SpA or ankylosing spondylitis) and spondyloarthropathy without radiographic changes in the sacro-iliac joints (non-radiographic SpA). Not all those affected by axial spondyloarthropathy are positive for HLA B 27 and inflammatory markers may not correlate well with disease activity. MRI scan of sacro-iliac joints may detect early signs of sacroiiitis not detected on plain radiograph. MRI lumbosacral spine may miss the sacro-iliac joints and may not have STIR-weighted images to detect bone oedema.[45,46]

34. Answer c

Prolactin is produced in the pituitary gland but extra-pituitary prolactin is produced in many sites such as the ovaries, mammary glands, endometrium and prostate. Prolactin was identified initially in the 1920s and 1930s as a lactogenic hormone but it has become associated since then with many other biological functions. Dopamine inhibits prolactin release. Oestrogens can cause hyperprolactinaemia, which is why high-oestrogen states such as pregnancy can be associated with high prolactin levels. Although chest wall trauma has been associated with hyperprolactinaemia, breast examination, ultrasound and mammography have not. Hyperprolactinaemia may also occur in renal failure and liver cirrhosis. Current guidelines recommend that blood can be taken for prolactin at any time of day. Most prolactin exists in the body in its monomeric form but some exists in other polymeric forms, with large molecules known as macroprolactin. This is though to be less biologically active but may account for up to 40% of measured prolactin results in those with raised prolactin levels. It is most commonly corrected for in laboratory measurements by mixing and incubating with polyethylene glycol (PEG) to quantify the amount of macroglobulin.[50]

35. Answer c

Sickle cell disease consists of a variation of genotypes which may have an influence on the clinical manifestations of the condition. Sickle cell disease is an autosomal recessive monogenic condition with two HbS genes required for sickle cell disease. Carriers of one HbS gene, known as sickle cell trait, usually avoid severe manifestations of the condition. However compound heterozygotes for HbS and another haemoglobin abnormality such as HbC, HbE or HbD or β-thalassaemia will have clinical manifestations but usually less severe than sickle cell disease. HbS-β thalasseamia[0] is an exception to this.

Those with sickle cell disease and α-thalassaemia usually have less severe haemolysis but more severe vaso-occlusive sickle cell complications.

HbF (fetal haemoglobin) peaks in mid-gestation and is usually <1% of total haemoglobin in a healthy 6 month old infant. HbF tends to be higher in those with sickle cell disease. There are certain regional genetic variations associated with higher HbF levels that have less severe sickle cell disease. HbF is excluded from HbS polymerisation and so can limit its effects.

Sickle cell trait is protective against severe malaria. However studies in Africa show that those with sickle cell disease contract malaria in the same manner as the general population but are at greater risk of death. Those affected by sickle cell disease are immunocompromised due to hyposplenism.[48]

36. Answer a

Smoking remains the main cause of chronic obstructive pulmonary disease and smoking cessation has the greatest impact on improving the natural history of the condition.[53]

37. Answer e

BCG should be given intradermally. Evidence of protection for BCG is stronger in young children than in adults and there is no data showing benefit in those over 35 years of age. BCG can be given with or at any interval before or after another live vaccine. However no further vaccines should be given in the BCG arm for three months due to risk of regional lymphadenitis. BCG is a live vaccination and is contraindicated in those with HIV.[55]

38. Answer d

IgA nephropathy most commonly presents with macroscopic haematuria, often after an upper respiratory infection ('synpharingitic') or physical exertion, or with incidental microscopic haematuria or proteinuria. It may less commonly present with acute kidney injury. It can present at any age but peak incidence is in the second and third decades of life. 30-40% develop a progressive renal disease. The disease burden is greatest in east and south-east Asia where there is also a more aggressive form of disease. Best treatment is contentious but involves supportive treatment such as blood pressure management, as well as renin-angiotensin blockade including with ACE inhibitors, and in some cases immunosuppression. Renal biopsy is required for definitive diagnosis, showing IgA deposition in the renal mesangium.[59,60]

39. Answer e

The aetiology of sarcoidosis remains a mystery. It is likely that a combination of genetic and environmental factors are involved. The highest incidence is in those of African origin, with Asians and Hispanics the least affected. It most commonly affects the lungs and mediastinal lymph nodes and the skin is the most common extra-thoracic site. Non-caseating granulomas are typical but not pathognomonic of sarcoidosis as they occur in other conditions. Diagnosis requires a compatible clinical presentation with non-caseating granulomas on biopsy and the exclusion of other possible causes of granulomatous inflammation. Corticosteroids are first-line in treatment and methotrexate is the best researched and most frequently used steroid-sparing agent.[61]

40. Answer b

Dermatomyositis is one of the idiopathic inflammatory myopathies and may be grouped with polymyositis, inclusion body myositis and necrotising myopathy. It may present with typical purple rash on the eyelids (heliotrope rash) and erythematous rash and variable papules on the extensor surfaces of the digits (Grotton papules) or other extensor surfaces (Grotton sign). Photosensitivity may occur. Symmetrical proximal muscle weakness is a hallmark clinical feature. Muscle enzymes such as CK are elevated and 80% are associated with positive autoantibodies, which may be myositis-specific or myositis-associated. Histopathological appearances of muscle biopsy vary between polymyositis and dermatomyositis suggesting a possible separate pathological process. Affected individuals have an increased risk of malignancy, including lung, cervical and ovarian cancers.[62,63]

41. Answer b

The cardiac troponin complex is a component of the thin filament and plays a role in myocardial contraction. Troponin I and troponin T are specific for myocardium and troponin C also exists in skeletal muscle. Therefore troponin I and T are used in the assessment of acute coronary syndrome and are sensitive and specific for detecting myocardial damage. Troponin T does have a diurnal variation (peaking in the morning and reducing during the day with a night-time rise) but this does not appear to affect its diagnostic accuracy. Abnormal troponin testing has also been shown to be a negative prognostic factor in non-ST elevation acute coronary syndrome.[66]

42. Answer d

Syphilis is a bacterial infection caused by the spirochete Treponema pallidum. It infects only humans and there is no animal reservoir. It is mainly a sexually-transmitted disease but may be spread via blood products, needle-sharing or vertically through the placenta. Primary syphilis typically presents with a painless genital chancre but this ulceration may present in other areas such as the anal or oral areas. Syphilis is infectious in its primary and secondary phases as well as the early latent phase. It remains sensitive to penicillin.[69,70]

43. Answer a

Insulinoma is the most common cause of hypoglycaemia due to endogenous hyperinsulinaemia. 90% are benign, 90% are solitary, >90% occur at intrapancreatic sites and 90% are less than 2cm in diameter. It may present with neuroglycopenic symptoms such as confusion, behavioural change, seizures or coma. It can be screened for using Whipple's triad: 1. Symptoms of hypoglycaemia 2. Documented hypoglycaemia during symptoms 3. Resolution of symptoms on correction of glucose. Prolonged fasting for 72 hours is the gold standard for diagnosis and detects 99% of insulinomas, by measuring levels of insulin, C-peptide and proinsulin. Routinely measured insulin levels may be normal and the release of insulin may be pulsatile, leading to intermittent symptoms. First line treatment is surgical removal and involves pre-operative detection of the tumour which may require invasive techniques such as endoscopic ultrasound. It may occur in MEN I syndrome.[71,72]

44. Answer c

A lung nodule as detected radiologically is defined as a well-defined rounded opacity measuring up to 3cm in diameter. An opacity larger than 3cm is defined as a lung mass and has a different management pathway.[76]

45. Answer d

Mitral regurgitation is the most common valvular heart disease.[77]

46. Answer b

The 2009 'swine flu' epidemic was caused by influenza A (H1N1). Influenza A virus can acquire adaptive changes known as antigenic drift which can affect its ability to cause severe illness in humans There is a huge zoonotic reservoir and with this the possibility of jumping from animals to humans leading to a pandemic. Influenza A can be subdivided into different variants of its surface proteins hemagglutinin (HA) and neuraminidase (NA).

Influenza A (H5N1) caused the 'bird flu' outbreak in 1997. Influenza A (H3N2) caused the 'Hong Kong flu' pandemic in 1968. Influenza A (H2N2) caused the 'Asian flu' pandemic in 1957. Influenza A (H3N8) caused the 1889 pandemic of 'Russian flu'.[79]

47. Answer c

ANCA-associated vasculitis primarily affects small and medium-sized vessels. It can be subdivided into granulomatosis with polyangiitis (GPA, formerly Wegener's granulomatosis), microscopic polyangiitis, and eosinophilic granulomatosis with polyangiitis (EGPA). Anti-neutrophil cytoplasmic antibodies (ANCA) are usually positive, targeting either proteinase 3 (PR3-ANCA positive) or myeloperoxidase (MPO-ANCA). Sinonasal, pulmonary and musculoskeletal manifestations are the most common, and renal involvement can progress to end stage renal failure. Other manifestations include sensorineural hearing loss, mononeuritis multiplex, scleritis and gangrene. The manifestations of the disease range from mild to severe. Severe disease is fatal when untreated. Current treatment regimes with immunosuppressants involve inducing remission and then maintenance treatment regimes. Excess mortality remains even with treatment.[80]

48. Answer c

Bowen's disease refers to dysplastic atypical keratinocytes in the epidermis which have not breached the basement membrane. It is a premalignant lesion also known as squamous cell carcinoma in situ. Estimates of progression to squamous cell carcinoma range from 3 to 16% of lesions, with high risk lesions on the ear, nose, lip, or eyelid or lesions with a diameter of over 10 mm. The lesions are well demarcated, erythematous, non-itchy patches of plaques on sun-exposed sites. They are slow growing over years, with more rapidly growing lesions over weeks to months raising the suspicion of a malignant lesion. Atypical features such as ulceration should also raise the suspicion of malignancy.[81]

47. Answer e

Acute respiratory distress syndrome is a syndrome characterised by acute non-cardiogenic pulmonary oedema, hypoxaemia and the requirement for mechanical ventilation. There are many possible causes including pulmonary infection, sepsis, trauma, acute abdominal causes, near-drowning and aspiration of gastric contents, among other causes. Mortality rate has been described as 30-40%. It is a heterogenous condition and there is no known intervention as yet that changes the course of the illness, other than treatment of the underlying cause and supportive treatments.

Studies on steroid use in ARDS have been conflicting without a clear consensus emerging and are not recommended at present, but are used in some cases. ARDS can be classified into mild, moderate and severe depending on level of hypoxaemia.[82]

48. Answer c

Bowen's disease refers to dysplastic atypical keratinocytes in the epidermis which have not breached the basement membrane. It is a premalignant lesion also known as squamous cell carcinoma in situ. Estimates of progression to squamous cell carcinoma range from 3 to 16% of lesions, with high risk lesions on the ear, nose, lip, or eyelid or lesions with a diameter of over 10 mm. The lesions are well demarcated, erythematous, non-itchy patches of plaques on sun-exposed sites. They are slow growing over years, with more rapidly growing lesions over weeks to months raising the suspicion of a malignant lesion. Atypical features such as ulceration should also raise the suspicion of malignancy.[81]

49. Answer e

Acute respiratory distress syndrome is a syndrome characterised by acute non-cardiogenic pulmonary oedema, hypoxaemia and the requirement for mechanical ventilation. There are many possible causes including pulmonary infection, sepsis, trauma, acute abdomina causes, near-drowning and aspiration of gastric contents, among other causes. Mortality rate has been described as 30-40%. It is a heterogenous condition and there is no known intervention as yet that changes the course of the illness, other than treatment of the underlying cause and supportive treatments. Studies on steroid use in ARDS have been conflicting without a clear consensus emerging and are not recommended at present, but are used in some cases. ARDS can be classified into mild, moderate and severe depending on level of hypoxaemia.[82]

50. Answer e

Fanconi anaemia is an inherited chromosomal instab lity disorder characterised by a variation of physical manifestations and pancytopenia. It may be inherited as autosomal recessive, dominant or X -linked. There is a wide variation in its phenotype. 75% will have the physical manifestations such as short stature, abnormal skin pigmentation, limb deformities and microcephaly, among other features. Pancytopenia may present at any age, but often presents in the first decade. There is a several hundred-fold increased risk of acute myelogenous leukaemia and solid tumours such as HPV-associated head and neck and urogenitary cancers, among others. Androgens can be used to increase blood counts. Haematopoietic stem cell transplantation is the only curative treatment.[83,84]

Fanconi syndrome is an inherited or acquired disorder of renal proximal tubular function.[23]

51. Answer a

In descending order, the most common benign liver lesions are hepatic haemangioma, focal nodular hyperplasia and hepatic adenoma. They are more common in women in particularly those who use exogenous oestrogens. Contraception may need to be stopped in some women to prevent enlargement of lesions. Most will not require surveillance For example smaller lesions in an individual without liver cirrhosis will not require surveillance once there is some diagnostic certainty regarding the nature of the lesion. Hepatic adenomas may undergo malignant transformation and larger lesions are at risk of haemorrhage.[88]

52. Answer c

Neurocysticercosis is caused by infection of the neurological system by the larval stage of the tapeworm Taenia solium. Only humans and pigs host the tapeworm, and it is contracted by humans through undercooked pork products or by human to human spread via the faecal-oral route. It is endemic in the developing world and is a common cause of adult-onset epilepsy in affected countries. Taenia solium larvae (cysticercus) can remain viable for years and cause an inflammatory reaction when they degenerate. Infection may be completely asymptomatic. Lesions affecting the brain parenchyma may present with seizures which usually respond well to anti epileptic medications, but disease severity depends on the extent of the lesions. Extensive or calcified cysts can lead to intractable epilepsy. Subarachnoid and intraventricular disease is associated with significant morbidity and mortality. Almost any neurological presentation may occur and any centrally caused neurological deficit may manifest, but seizures are the most common presentation. Treatment with anti-parasitic agents such as albendazole can be effective but may worsen symptoms by causing inflammation, so seizures should be controlled initially prior to starting any anti-parasitic treatment. Treatment involves a combination of anti-parasitic agents, steroids, management of seizures and other neurological manifestations, and neurosurgical intervention where necessary.[89]

53. Answer a

Although the pathophysiology of multiple sclerosis is not fully understood, it is known to manifest as inflammatory central nervous system lesions disseminated in space and time. Relapsing-remitting multiple sclerosis comprises 85% of cases and current treatments can prevent relapses and disability to an extent in this type. A clinically isolated syndrome is a monophasic clinical episode with patient-reported symptoms and objective findings reflecting a focal or multifocal inflammatory demyelinating event in the CNS, developing acutely or subacutely, with a duration of at least 24 h, with or without recovery, and in the absence of fever or infection, similar to a typical multiple sclerosis relapse (attack and exacerbation) but in a patient not known to have multiple sclerosis. Bilateral optic neuritis is an atypical presentation for multiple sclerosis, with unilateral optic neuritis more common. In a patient presenting with unilateral optic neuritis this would constitute a clinically isolated syndrome requiring use of the McDonald criteria to assess if multiple sclerosis can be diagnosed. MRI findings without clinical symptoms or signs cannot diagnose multiple sclerosis although may constitute a radiologically isolated syndrome.[90,91]

54. Answer c

Nikolsky sign occurs in Stevens Johnson syndrome, where bullae come away from the underlying skin when lightly rubbed.[92]

55. Answer d

Corticosteroids can be classified as predominantly glucocorticoid (involved in carbohydrate metabolism) or mineralocorticoid (involved in fluid and electrolyte balance) although many corticosteroids have both properties. Glucocorticoid activity is closely related to anti-inflammatory potency, the main therapeutic indication for corticosteroids. Synthetic steroids were originally developed to maximise anti-inflammatory potency, with dexamethasone 25 times more potent than cortisol.[93]

56. Answer b

Severe acute respiratory syndrome (SARS) emerged as a condition in 2002 when a novel coronavirus, SARS-CoV, caused an outbreak of atypical pneumonia in China and Hong Kong. Adult respiratory distress syndrome (ARDS) refers to a severe lung condition characterised by hypoxaemia, non cardiogenic pulmonary oedema and the requirement for ventilation with pneumonia just one of many possible causes. Fever, cough and myalgia are common presenting symptoms in SARS CoV infection, with rhinorrhoea less frequent. Absolute lymphopenia was found in 98% of SARS-CoV infections. Infection in children and teenagers is usually mild with the elderly more at risk of severe disease. Nosocomial spread predominated in the original SARS outbreak in 2002-2003 with community spread less common. Droplet spread via the respiratory route is the primary form of spread although spread via other environmental pathways as well as the faecal oral route is postulated.[94]

57. Answer b

Cephalosporins and penicillins share a similar central four-membered betalactam ring, with variations in molecules being conferred by their side chains. It was originally thought that 10% of those with penicillin allergy were allergic to cephalosporins, but further study has cast doubt on this number. Cephalosporin allergy is uncommon (1-3% of the population) with cephalosporin-induced anaphylaxis estimated at 0.0001-0.1% of the population. Cephalosporins are broad-spectrum antibiotics. There are six generations of cephalosporins, and each generation has a different allergy risk, varying depending on its R1 side chain. Allergy to one generation does not imply allergy to another. First and second generation cephalosporins may have increased risk of being allergenic in those with penicillin allergy with newer studies suggesting cross-reactivity of 2-5%, with studies showing other cephalosporins having little or no increased risk. Also those who have a known drug allergy in general are at increased risk of another so this may be a factor in any cross-reactivity.[95]

58. Answer a

Drug reaction with eosinophilia and systemic symptoms (DRESS syndrome) is an uncommon drug hypersensitivity reaction. It tends to present with widespread rash, facial oedema, fever, lymphadenopathy and variable visceral involvement. It typically presents within 2 to 6 weeks of drug exposure and can affect any age. Morbilliform rash is the most common skin manifestation although urticaria, erythema multiforme or pustular rash may occur. Liver dysfunction is the most common non-dermatological manifestation and may present as either a hepatocellular or cholestatic picture. Myocarditis may be initially asymptomatic and may present up to 4 months after initial presentation. DRESS syndrome is associated with a delayed presentation of separate autoimmune conditions with autoimmune thyroiditis the most common.[97]

59. Answer c

Methotrexate is a folate antagonist which inhibits the synthesis of purine and pyrimidine rings in DNA. It is primarily excreted by the renal route. Subcutaneous methotrexate has been shown to have greater efficacy in some conditions and oral methotrexate is usually better tolerated. It was originally developed as an anti-cancer agent and is a first-line disease modifying agent in many rheumatological conditions. How exactly it exerts its anti-inflammatory effects in rheumatological conditions is not known, but the finding that folate supplementation does not reduce its anti-inflammatory effects suggests that there may be an alternative mechanism to folate antagonism. It is given in a weekly dosage.[98]

60. Answer e

Primary ciliary dyskinesia (PCD) is an autosomal recessive disorder with heterogenous genotypes and phenotypes. It typically presents in early childhood with neonatal respiratory distress, oto-rhino-sinus disease and chronic productive cough. Male infertility occurs due to abnormal sperm motility. Cystic fibrosis is an important differential diagnosis and must be excluded. The triad of chronic sinusitis, bronchiectasis and situs inversus is known as Kartagener syndrome. The presentation is variable, with several potential genetic mutations affecting varying aspects of ciliary function. Organ laterality defects occur in about 50% of cases.

Diagnosis is challenging, using a combination of clinical presentation, epithelial biopsies (may be structurally and functionally normal) and nasal nitric oxide (reduced in those with PCD). Nasal saccharine clearance testing has not been validated. Advances in genetic testing has also become more useful in aiding diagnosis. Bronchiectasis may present in childhood and is present in all adults with PCD.[99]

61. Answer c

The components of the CHA_2DS_2 -VASc score are congestive heart failure/ left ventricular dysfunction, hypertension, age (> 75 years for 2 points and 65 to 74 years for 1 point), diabetes mellitus, previous stroke/TIA, vascular disease and sex category (female).[102]

62. Answer a

Cutaneous T cell lymphoma is an extranodal form of non-Hodgkins lymphoma involving infiltration of the skin by monoclonal malignant T cells. These conditions can be very difficult to diagnose due their non-specific presentation, often mimicking benign skin conditions. The most common is mycosis fungoides. Its leukaemic variant is known as Sezary syndrome. These are incurable conditions and tend to relapse after stopping treatment, so management is palliative. LDH levels can be useful to indicate tumour burden but are non-specific. Treatment involves a combination of topical and systemic treatment to slow the progression of disease.[103]

63. Answer c

Parkinson's disease is a neurodegenerative condition characterized by rest tremor, muscle rigidity, slowed movement (bradykinesia), and often postural instability.[104]

64. Answer c

There is an increased risk of coeliac disease associated with many autoimmune conditions, as well as chromosomal disorders such as Down's syndrome, William's syndrome and Turner's syndrome. There is an increased risk with type 1 diabetes but not type 2 diabetes.[105]

65. Answer c

Lipomas are benign tumours of fat cells (adipocytes). They are more common in individuals with diabetes mellitus and hyperlipidaemia. They are usually 2-3 cm diameter but may be much larger. They are painless and mobile. Multiple lipomas are seen in 5-10% of cases and are associated with certain genetic conditions such as familial lipomatosis. They are usually best left alone unless there is concern about malignancy such as liposarcoma.[106]

66. Answer d

Non-alcoholic fatty liver disease (NAFLD) is increasingly common. It is predominantly a diagnosis of exclusion by ruling out other causes of liver steatosis. Previously thought to be a benign condition NAFLD is now seen as a disease that can lead to liver fibrosis and cirrhosis. The level of liver fibrosis is the main way of determining risk of progression. Liver ultrasound has good sensitivity and specificity for detecting steatosis (85% and 95% respectively) but is not good at detecting fibrosis. Other radiological measures such as Fibroscan (liver stiffness measurements assessed with transient elastography) are better at detecting fibrosis. Liver biopsy is the best way of detecting steatosis and fibrosis but has some risks and may be normal in a patchy disease and is not usually necessary in NAFLD.[107,108]

67. Answer e

Non-secreting pituitary adenomas typically present with local compression signs such as headaches or visual disturbance, typically bitemporal hemianopia or reduced visual acuity. Two thirds present with reduced gonadotropin levels and signs of hypogonadism. Raised gonadotropin levels are rare. 10% present with pituitary apoplexy with sudden onset retro-orbital pain and sudden onset visual disturbance or loss. Surgical resection with or without radiotherapy is the usual choice of treatment. Complete resection is achieved in 65% of patients, with resolution of visual deficits in 80%. Recurrence largely depends on the invasiveness of the tumour.[109]

68. Answer d

The Rinne test involves placing the base of a 512 Hz tuning fork at the mastoid process and then one inch from the external auditory meatus. A Rinne negative is when the tuning fork is not heard at the external meatus after being held against the mastoid process, implying that bone conduction is greater than air conduction and that there is a conductive hearing deficit in that ear. There may be a false negative if there is a profound sensorineural deafness in that ear and the sound is being heard by the other ear, and this can be overcome by masking the other ear with white noise. A true Rinne negative test requires a hearing loss of at least 20 decibels.[110]

69. Answer b

Phocomelia refers to shortened limbs arising in the children of pregnant women due to exposure to thalidomide.[113]

70. Answer c

Q fever is caused by the bacterium Coxiella burnetti. The bacterium does not produce spores but forms a spore-like state once in the outside environment and can survive for years. Early antibiotic treatment with doxycycline is important to prevent chronic infection which can be severe and has a high mortality rate. It can be spread from sheep, cattle and goats. Francisella tularensis caused tularaemia.[114]

71. Answer a

Chronic atrophic gastritis (CAG) is a chronic disease whose main features are atrophy or metaplasia of gastric glands. It may be autoimmune or associated with Helicobacter pylori infection. Whether these factors interact to cause CAG or whether they are two distinct entities is uncertain. CAG can present with microcytic anaemia due to iron deficiency or macrocytic anaemia due to vitamin B12 deficiency. As a result of gastric gland destruction in advanced disease there is achlorhydria (reduced gastric acid secretion). There is an association with other autoimmune diseases including type 1 diabetes mellitus. CAG is seen as a pre-malignant lesion with increased risk of intestinal type gastric cancer and gastric carcinoid.[115,116,117]

72. Answer d

The IARC classifies substances as group1 (known carcinogens), group 2a (probable carcinogens), group 2b (possible carcinogens) and group 3 (not classifiable). The classification reflects the level of available evidence and not necessarily the actual cancer risk.[118]

73. Answer e

Hidradenitis suppurativa is a chronic inflammatory skin condition characterised by painful subcutaneous nodules. Its exact pathogenesis is uncertain. It is more common in those with negative metabolic factors such as insulin resistance, obesity and smoking. About a third of those affected have a positive family history with an autosomal dominant pattern of inheritance. Increased incidence has also been found n certain autoimmune conditions such as spondyloarthopathies.[119]

74. Answer d

A review of oseltamivir for the treatment of influenza was published in 2014 after obtaining clinical study reports from the drug manufacturers and documentation from regulators. Clinical study reports are given by drug companies to regulators during the process of obtaining licencing for a drug and may run to thousands of pages. A published clinical paper is a succinct summary of this data. On review of these reports the author of this review concluded that there was no evidence that oseltamivir or zanamivir, another neuraminidase inhibitor, reduced the rate of hospita isation or influenza complications. There is evidence that it improves recovery from influenza by 16.8 hours on average. This refuted previous conclusions where the efficacy of oseltamivir may have been overestimated by published industry-sponsored studies. Oseltamivir is taken orally and zanamivir is inhaled.[121]

75. Answer a

80% of primary hyperparathyroidism occurs due to a single adenoma, with less than 10% occurring due to hyperplasia of all four glands and 1% due to parathyroid carcinoma. There is increased risk of reduced bone mineral density and osteoporosis compared with the general population and increased risk of fractures of the spine, forearm, ribs and pelvis have been demonstrated. However it is less clear whether there is an increased risk of hip fracture. The distal radius seems particularly sensitive to reduced mineral density in primary hyperparathyroidism. Hypocalcaemia due to malabsorption in inflammatory bowel disease would be secondary hyperparathyroidism.[122]

76. Answer a

Available evidence on long-term macrolide use suggests possible improvement in symptom control and rescue-inhaler use, but not in other measured parameters. Studies are relatively small and do not currently suggest a role for long-term macrolide use in asthma.[123]

77. Answer b

The most common sustained arrhythmia is atrial fibrillation.[124]

78. Answer e

SARS CoV-2 is an RNA virus. It enters human cells through the angiotensin converter enzyme-2 (ACE-2) receptor. The most common mode of transmission is via droplet spread but other modes of transmission such as aerosol spread are thought possible. It is usually diagnosed via reverse transcriptase polymerase chain reaction (RT-PCR) of a swab, most commonly nasopharyngeal swab.[125]

79. Answer a

Bechet's disease is a chronic inflammatory vasculitis affecting multiple organ systems with features of both an autoimmune and autoinflammatory condition. The peak age of presentation is 18 to 40 years and it rarely presents over the age of 55. Vasculitis can affect both venous and arterial vessels. Venous thrombosis occurs in 30% of cases. Oral ulceration is indistinguishable from aphthous ulceration and is painful, with scarring genital ulceration also common. Other cutaneous manifestations such as erythema nodosum and pseudofolliculitis also occur. Sight-threatening ocular involvement is common with posterior uveitis a common feature.[126]

80. Answer e

Those with diabetes between age 40 and 75 with a raised LDL above 70mg/dl (1.8mmol/l) should be commenced on a statin and do not need an assessment of 10 year cardiovascular risk, according to the American College of Cardiology–American Heart Association (ACC–AHA) guidelines on cholesterol management and prevention of cardovascular disease. Statins inhibit f 3-hydroxy-3-methylglutaryl coenzyme A (HMG-CoA) reductase which leads to increased expression of the hepatic LDL receptor and increased clearance of LDL from the circulation. Long term statin use may increase the risk of developing diabetes by 0.2% per year. The benefits of statin use are greater in the second, third, and fourth years than in the first year. Ezetimibe has not been shown to improve cardiovascular outcomes when used in isolation. There is evidence of its benefit in those after acute myocardial infarction when added to statin treatment. [127]

81. Answer a

The most common genetic mutation in haemochromatosis is a G-to-A missense mutation leading to the substitution of tyrosine for cysteine at amino acid position 282 of the protein product (C282Y). Because of variable penetrance of the genetic mutations involved in haemochromatosis, homozygosity may not necessarily reflect subsequent iron overload requiring treatment. Estimates vary as regards how many homozygous or compound heterozygotes will develop phenotypic haemochromatosis. First degree relatives of an affected individual should have iron study testing as well as genetic testing. Transferrin saturation is calculated by the equation:

Serum iron/total iron binding capacity x 100

and reflects the saturation of the body's iron binding capacity.

Removal of 500mls of blood removes 250mg of iron.[128]

82. Answer b

Hodgkin's lymphoma is a malignancy arising from germinal centre and post-germinal centre B cells. It is characterised by the presence of multinucleate giant cells or large mononuclear cells known as Hodgkin and Reed Sternberg (HRS) cells. Hodgkin's lymphoma is subdivided into classical Hodgkin's lymphoma (cHL) accounting for 90% of cases, and nodular lymphocyte predominant Hodgkin's lymphoma (NLPHL).

NLHPL has a more indolent course in general than cHL. cHL itself is subdivided into four categories according to its histological appearance and predominance of Hodgkin and Reed Sternberg (HRS) cells and inflammatory background:

- Nodular sclerosing (NSCHL): the most common accounting for 70% of cases, it is more likely to present with mediastinal adenopathy and has a better prognosis than other subtypes
- Mixed cellularity (MCCHL): accounting for 20-25% of cases, it is more common in those with HIV and in the developing world and has a stronger association with Epstein Barr virus than NSCHL. Along with LDCHL tends to have a worse prognosis than NSCHL and LRCHL.
- Lymphocyte rich (LRCHL): more likely to present with peripheral adenopathy than bulky mediastinal adenopathy and has an excellent prognosis
- Lymphocyte depleted (LDCHL): comprises <1% of cHL, it has an association with HIV infection and a poor prognosis[129,130]

83. Answer b

Crohn's disease is a chronic inflammatory condition of the gastrointestinal tract with frequent extraintestinal manifestations. It is believed to be caused by a combination of genetic and environmental factors. Increased risk of developing the disease has been associated with smoking, use of oral contraceptives, antibiotics and non-steroidal inflammatory medications. Homozygosity for the NOD 2 gene has been associated with a 20 to 40-fold increased risk of developing the disease. Vaccines have not been shown to increase risk.[131]

84. Answer b

Propranolol reduces circulating serum T_3 levels in a dose dependent manner. It has no effect on other thyroid hormone levels. It is used in hyperthyroidism because of its nonselective betablocker properties which reduces symptoms such as tremor and anxiety, and also its effect on T_3 which may be reduced by 20-30% depending on dose.[134]

85. Answer d

Obstructive sleep apnoea (OSA) is characterized by partial (hypopnea) or complete (apnoea) collapse of the upper airways during sleep, causing intermittent hypoxemia and sleep fragmentation. It is a significant cause of increased morbidity and mortality as well as a cause of occupational accidents, in particular road traffic accidents in commercial drivers. It is often asymptomatic or symptoms may be under-reported. The apnoea-hypopnea index (AHI) measures the number of events per hour of sleep and is classed as mild (5 – 14), moderate (15-30) and severe (>30). Good adherence to CPAP treatment is indicated by use of the machine for at least 4 hours per night 70% of the time. OSA has been shown to increase the risk of road traffic accidents by a factor of 2 to 5. Good adherence to treatment has been shown to reduce the accident rate to that of the general population. Poor adherence to treatment has been shown to be ineffective in reducing accident rates. Obesity increases risk but it does occur in the non-obese, with functional and anatomical factors important in its pathogenesis.[132,133]

86. Answer c

D Dimer is a biomarker of fibrin activity and degradation and serves as an indirect marker of thrombotic activity. It has been mostly used in exclusion of venous thromboembolic disease to try and avoid costly radiological testing. There is large variation among different assays used, with high sensitivity tests having relatively low specificity. It is most useful in excluding venous thromboembolic disease where the pre-test probability is low. D Dimer levels increase with advancing age, in those with cancer and after trauma, immobilisation and surgery. Levels progressively increase during a normal pregnancy. The test is less useful where the pre-test probability is high when radiology should be considered. A positive D Dimer test taken one month after finishing anti-coagulation has been shown to be associated with a higher risk of recurrence, especially in men, so D Dimer testing may have a limited role in deciding on duration of anticoagulation in selected patients. A negative test is sufficient to exclude disseminated intravascular coagulation, but the test lacks specificity so is insufficient for diagnosis.[135]

87. Answer c

Harlequin syndrome occurs due to unilateral facial sympathetic denervation with compensatory excessive flushing and sweating of the contralateral side in certain situations such as exertion. It is a benign condition. The term should only be used where an underlying cause cannot be identified, and if an underlying neurological cause is found then it should be termed Harlequin sign. Possible causes of Harlequin sign are dissection of the carotid artery, toxic goitre, tumours, syringomyelia, multiple sclerosis, and iatrogenic effects of invasive procedures. Ptosis and anisocoria (unequal pupils) may be associated but are not necessary for diagnosis.[137]

88. Answer b

Ebola virus disease is caused by a filovirus species causing periodic outbreaks in humans in Africa since 1976. Filoviruses include the Ebola virus and Marburg virus species. They are filamentous RNA viruses. They are zoonotic pathogens and they are maintained in animal reservoirs.[138]

89. Answer c

Heart failure with preserved ejection fraction (HFpEF) is characterised by heart failure symptoms with a preserved ejection fraction of >50% as well as signs of diastolic dysfunction on echocardiography. These signs include concentric left ventricular hypertrophy and signs of increased left ventricular end diastolic pressure. NYHA symptoms must be present for diagnosis. BNP and NT-pro BNP are usually raised. A traditional pathophysiological model associated HFpEF with systemic hypertension and vascular dysfunction leading to left ventricular hypertrophy and reduced ventricular compliance causing diastolic dysfunction. An emerging pathophysiological model postulates that pro inflammatory states such as obesity, diabetes and hypertension lead to an inflammatory remodelling process of the left ventricle with results in a fibrosis and reduced compliance. Loop diuretics are shown to improve symptoms and quality of life but no medications have been shown to improve any endpoints such as mortality in HFpEF.[139]

90. Answer e

Necrotising fasciitis is an infection of the subcutanecus tissues and fascia. It can be difficult to differentiate clinically from other soft tissue infections. It is an emergency and requires a high index of suspicion to diagnose, as early surgical intervention improves outcome. It has a mortality of 20.6%. The most common site is the perineum but it can occur anywhere. It is a clinical diagnosis. A factor which may aid differentiation from other soft tissue infections is severe pain out of proportion to the level of skin involvement, often in adjacent normal skin. Signs of systemic illness such as fever and tachycardia, as well as signs of cutaneous necrosis and gas gangrene may indicate necrotising fasciitis, but these are late signs. CT scan has a high sensitivity and specificity for identifying signs of necrotising fasciitis and is the radiological modality of choice. However it is largely a clinical diagnosis and investigation should not delay appropriate resuscitation and urgent surgical referral for debridement.[140,141]

91. Answer c

A first degree relative with ulcerative colitis (UC) increases an individual's risk of UC four-fold. A history of previous smoking is one of the strongest risk factors for UC, with active smokers having lower risk than former or non-smokers. Urban living and NSAID use are associated with increased risk. Appendicectomy for acute appendicitis has a protective effect against developing UC.[142]

92. Answer b

Infective endocarditis (IE) is a multisystem disease arising from infection of the endocardium of the heart. Rheumatic fever has declined as a risk factor in the developed world, now accounting for 5% of cases although it remains the most common risk factor in the developing world. Degenerative heart disease is a more common risk factor now in the developed world. Prosthetic heart valves and cardiac devices as well as healthcare-acquired infection are also increasing in prevalence as risk factors for IE. IE is uniformly fatal if untreated and even with best treatment mortality is still 25%. IE caused by enterococci is associated with health care contact and is increasing in incidence, but remains less common than staphylococcal and streptococcal causes. Blood cultures are negative in 10% of cases, which may be due to recent antibiotic use or if caused by uncommon pathogens which are difficult to isolate. Infection rarely occurs in a normal endocardium, and some damage to the integrity of the heart is needed o allow thrombotic vegetations to develop.[143,]

93. Answer e

DPP-4 inhibitors reduce breakdown of incretins which are insulotropic enteroendocrine hormones produced in response to glucose intake. Examples are sitagliptin and linagliptin. Glucagon-like peptide-1 is an incretin and GLP-1 agonists enhance their action. Examples are liraglutide and exenatide.

Thiazolidinediones such as pioglitazone act by regulating peroxisome proliferator-activated receptor-gamma mediated gene expression resulting in increased insulin sensitivity and glucose utilization, and decreased glucose production.

SGLT-2 inhibitors such as dapagliflozin and empagliflozin improve glycaemic control by reducing glucose reabsorption in the renal proximal tubule resulting in glycosuria.[145]

94. Answer a
α-thalassaemia is a haemoglobinopathy caused by abnormal α chains in the haemoglobin molecule. There are over 100 genetic forms identified. α chains are produced by two genes on each chromosome but β chains come from a single gene locus. The severity depends on the number of non-functioning α globin genes. Defective production of α globin leads to excess β globin production of β chains in adults, which lead to β_4 tetramers known as haemoglobin H (HbH) which do not transport oxygen well due their high oxygen affinity. α-thalassaemia is protective against severe malaria which has led to its selective proliferation in tropical and subtropical regions. α^0-thalassaemia indicates inactivation of the two α globin genes on one chromosome (--/αα) and is more severe than the α^+-thalassaemia, which occurs when one of the two α globin genes on one chromosome are disabled (-α/αα).[146]

95. Answer c

Allogeneic hematopoietic cell transplantation (allo-HCT) has become an increasingly available treatment for incurable haematological conditions and the most common complication is graft vs host disease (GVHD). GVHD may be acute or chronic. It occurs when immunocompetent T cells from the donor recognise the recipient as foreign and trigger an immune reaction. Clinical signs of acute GVHD include a maculopapular rash, jaundice and hyperbilirubinaemia due to bile duct damage and gastrointestinal symptoms such as nausea, vomiting and bloody diarrhoea. Skin reactions are the first and most common presentation, followed by gastrointestinal signs and symptoms. Risk factors for GVHD include the degree of HLA mismatch, unrelated donors and female donor and male recipient among others. The reaction can be induced by major histocompatibility complex (MHC) or minor histocompatibility antigen (miH) disparities. Risk can be reduced by minimising disparities between donor and recipient, and immunosuppression regimes such as cyclosporin and methotrexate. First line treatment is with corticosteroids, and failure to respond to corticosteroids is a poor prognostic sign in GVHD.[148]

96. Answer d

Nutcracker syndrome results from compression of the left renal vein between the aorta and the superior mesenteric artery. It may occur in men and women. The peak prevalence is in young and middle aged adults but it may present at any age. It may cause renal angle or pelvic pain, visible or invisible haematuria, proteinuria and varicocele. It may require surgical intervention if symptoms are severe.[1]

97. Answer d

Transient ischaemic attack (TIA) involves transient neurological signs or symptoms usually lasting seconds to minutes and usually less than one hour, with no radiological signs of an acute ischaemic infarct on brain radiology. Investigations to find the source of an embolism is important, such as ECG, echocardiogram and radiology of neck arteries. However the preferred initial investigation in the acute setting for diagnosis and to guide further management is diffusion weighted imaging assessed with MRI scan.[150]

98. Answer a

The sensitivity of a test refers to the proportion of people with a condition who have a positive test result. It can be calculated as:

true positives/ (true positives + false negatives)

The proportion of people without a condition who have a negative test result is the specificity of a test.

The proportion of people with a condition who have a negative test result is the false negative rate.

The proportion of people without a condition who have a positive test result is the false positive rate.

The proportion of people with a condition with a given test result (either positive or negative) divided by the proportion of people without the condition with that result is the likelihood ratio.[151]

99. Answer d

Tumour lysis syndrome (TLS) is a biochemical complication of rapid cell breakdown associated with malignancy. It usually arises as a result of chemotherapy. It may occur spontaneously but this is rare. It can be subdivided into laboratory TLS or clinical TLS. Biochemical features of laboratory TLS are hyperkalaemia, hyperphosphataemia, hyperuricaemia and hypocalcaemia. Laboratory TLS does require treatment, with hyperkalaemia the most serious manifestation. Clinical TLS is laboratory TLS with clinical features which include acute kidney injury, seizures and cardiac arrhythmias or arrest. Acute kidney injury is the most common clinical manifestation, and hyperkalaemia is the earliest biochemical abnormality. TLS most commonly occurs with haematological malignancies such as lymphoma, leukaemia and multiple myeloma, but may occur after treatment for other malignancies.[152]

100. Answer b

Tetanus is a potentially fatal disease caused by a neurotoxin produced by clostridium tetani. Vaccination is highly protective and natural immunity does not occur. It is the only vaccine preventable non-communicable disease. Tetanus spores can remain viable for years and are present in the soil and intestines and faeces of many animals. The incubation period is 2 days to several months but most cases have developed within two weeks. The shorter the incubation period the greater the risk of death. Generalised tetanus starts usually with lockjaw and trismus and becomes more general-ised, and is more common than localised tetanus. Localised tetanus is un-common in humans and is characterised by localised muscle spasms in the area of a wound. Metronidazole is included in the treatment regimen. At-tempts to culture the organism are usually unsuccessful and the diagnosis is clinical.[153]

1. The most common symptom in aortic stenosis is:
   a.   Exertional syncope
   b.   Collapse
   c.   Dyspnoea
   d.   Exertional chest pain
   e.   Palpitations

2. Food-bound cobalamin malabsorption (FBCM):
   a.   Causes fewer cases of vitamin B12 deficiency than pernicious anaemia
   b.   May be associated with proton pump inhibitor use
   c.   May be associated with sulphonylurea use
   d.   Requires intramuscular vitamin B12 replacement
   e.   Does not lead to neurological manifestations of vitamin B12 deficiency

3. The following is the appropriate sequence for virus type with regard to the following: HIV - hepatitis C - hepatitis B:
   a.   Retrovirus – RNA virus – DNA virus
   b.   RNA virus -retrovirus – DNA virus
   c.   Retrovirus -DNA virus – RNA virus
   d.   RNA virus – DNA virus – retrovirus
   e.   DNA virus – RNA virus – retrovirus

4. Acute urticaria:
   a.   Will not progress to anaphylaxis
   b.   May be induced by external pressure
   c.   Avoidance of certain foods may be necessary in treatment
   d.   Usually has a clearly defined trigger
   e.   May cause scarring of the skin

5. The gold standard for malaria diagnosis is:
- a. Light microscopy of Giemsa stained blood-smear
- b. Polymerase chain reaction of parasitic nucleic acid
- c. ELISA testing for parasitic antibodies
- d. Rapid diagnostic testing for parasitic antigens
- e. It is a clinical diagnosis

6. Alpha-1 antitrypsin deficiency:
- a. Is inherited in an autosomal dominant manner
- b. The PiMM genotype indicates the most severe form of disease
- c. All non-smokers will develop lung disease
- d. Does not manifest clinically in childhood
- e. Alpha-1 antitrypsin may act as an acute phase reactant

7. The most common cause of blindness worldwide is:
- a. Diabetes
- b. Trachoma
- c. Cataract
- d. Onchocerciasis
- e. CMV retinitis

8. Chronic obstructive pulmonary disease (COPD):
- a. Will not progress once smoking is stopped
- b. The GOLD guidelines classify COPD according to lung function, patient-reported symptoms and exacerbations
- c. Long term macrolide antibiotics slow progression of the disease
- d. Inhaled corticosteroids are contraindicated in COPD
- e. The benefits of pulmonary rehabilitation have not been shown to exceed the benefits of pharmacological management in COPD

9. Which of the following is <u>not</u> a known non-cardiac cause of a rise in natriuretic peptides:
   a. Older age
   b. Renal impairment
   c. Systemic bacterial infection
   d. Obesity
   e. Female gender

10. Primary adrenal insufficiency (PAI):
   a. Is most commonly caused by long-term steroid therapy
   b. May require dynamic testing for diagnosis
   c. Oral dexamethasone is the replacement treatment of choice
   d. Oral steroid replacement therapy should be given twice daily with the higher dose in the evening to mimic natural diurnal variation
   e. Replacement therapy should be monitored by checking ACTH and cortisol levels

11. Primary mitral regurgitation:
   a. The direction of radiation of the murmur can help identify the valvular leaflet involved.
   b. Will rarely progress to heart failure
   c. Outcome is unrelated to symptoms
   d. Operative intervention is indicated only when an individual is symptomatic
   e. Mitral valve replacement is associated with lower mortality and fewer complication than mitral valve repair

12. The commonest technique for lab detection of respiratory viruses is:
   a. Viral culture
   b. Direct immunofluorescence
   c. Light microscopy
   d. Polymerase chain reaction (PCR)
   e. Point of care testing

13. The most commonly involved mucosal site in Stevens Johnson syndrome and toxic epidermal necrolysis (SJS/TEN) is:
    a. Mouth
    b. Eyes
    c. Nose
    d. Genital area
    e. Large bowel

14. Adverse effects to methotrexate are most commonly:
    a. Gastrointestinal
    b. Renal
    c. Haematological
    d. Musculoskeletal
    e. Respiratory

15. Pectus excavatum:
    a. Accounts for 50% of all chest deformities
    b. Is usually associated with an underlying connective tissue disorder
    c. In affected individuals it is always evident in the newborn period
    d. May cause cardiorespiratory compromise
    e. Affects males and females equally

16. Atrial fibrillation:
    a. Atrial fibrillation with valvular heart disease (as opposed to non-valvular atrial fibrillation) refers to atrial fibrillation associated with rheumatic mitral valve stenosis or mechanical prosthetic valve
    b. Direct oral anti coagulants are preferable to vitamin K antagonists for stroke prevention in valvular atrial fibrillation
    c. Risk of stroke is less in valvular atrial fibrillation than in non-valvular atrial fibrillation
    d. Thrombus is more likely to occur in the left atrium in valvular atrial fibrillation than in non-valvular atrial fibrillation
    e. Direct oral anti coagulants are inferior to warfarin for stroke prevention in atrial fibrillation associated with aortic stenosis

17. Serology in coeliac disease:
a. Anti-transglutaminase antibodies (tTG antibodies) are IgA antibodies
b. Anti-transglutaminase antibodies (tTG antibodies) are IgG antibodies
c. Anti-endomysium antibodies (EmA antibodies) are more sensitive than anti-transglutaminase antibodies (tTG antibodies)
d. IgA DGP antibodies (direct antibodies against deaminated gliadin peptides) are useful in diagnosing adults with coeliac disease
e. The reduction of tTG antibodies with a gluten free diet reflects regrowth of intestinal villi

18. Acromegaly:
a. Increased mortality is most commonly from pressure effects of the adenoma
b. Is usually caused by a non-invasive adenoma
c. Does not require dynamic testing for diagnosis
d. Obstructive sleep apnoea is a common association
e. Does not respond to dopamine agonist treatment

19. Helicobacter pylori:
a. Is a gram-positive bacterium
b. Cannot survive in an acidic environment
c. Is not sensitive to penicillin
d. Is a group 1 carcinogen as classified by the International Agency for Research on Cancer
e. Does not need eradication in asymptomatic individuals

20. Pityriasis rosea:
a. Is triggered by herpes zoster virus
b. More commonly occurs on the limbs than on the trunk
c. Will not relapse
d. Persistence beyond 12 weeks excludes the diagnosis
e. May be associated with increased risk of miscarriage in pregnancy

21. Exacerbations in chronic obstructive pulmonary disease:
    a. Do not affect mortality
    b. Do not affect progression of the disease
    c. Do not affect underlying health status
    d. The frequency and severity of exacerbations is associated with long-term mortality independent of comorbidities, FEV1, age and body mass index
    e. Are not reduced with long-term antibiotic therapy

22. Which if the following is the most accurate with regard to flecainide:
    a. It has a positive inotropic effect
    b. It prolongs the QT interval
    c. It is safe to use in heart failure
    d. It should not be used in a structurally abnormal heart
    e. It is not effective for converting acute atrial fibrillation to sinus rhythm

23. Which of the following is not a typical feature of COVID 19:
    a. Lymphocytosis
    b. Elevated CRP
    c. Elevated D Dimer
    d. Elevated LDH
    e. Ground glass shadowing on CXR

24. Hodgkin's lymphoma:
    a. Malignant cells make up the majority of the tumour
    b. Arises from T cells
    c. Accounts for the majority of lymphoma diagnoses
    d. Immunosuppression is a risk factor
    e. Requires the presence of Epstein Barr virus for diagnosis

25. The most common areas of the gastrointestinal tract affected in an individual with Crohn's disease are:
    a. Ileum and colon
    b. Perianal area only
    c. Colon only
    d. Small bowel only
    e. Gastroduodenal region

26. Amiodarone and thyroid abnormalities:
    a. A 200mg amiodarone tablet contains 500 times the recommended daily allowance of iodine
    b. Most of those on amiodarone will develop thyroid abnormalities
    c. Amiodarone-induced hypothyroidism is more likely to occur in iodine-deficient areas
    d. Amiodarone induced hyperthyroidism will resolve within one week of ceasing the medication
    e. Replacement thyroid hormone can always be stopped once amiodarone is stopped in amiodarone induced hypothyroidism

27. The most common form of primary immunodeficiency is:
    a. Common variable immunodeficiency
    b. Severe combined immunodeficiency
    c. Natural killer cell deficiency
    d. Autoinflammatory disorders
    e. Complement deficiency

28. The most common presenting symptom in ulcerative colitis is:
    a. Rectal bleeding
    b. Abdominal pain
    c. Fever
    d. Weight loss
    e. Vomiting

29. Which if the following is not a common presenting symptom of COVID 19 within the first 5 days of illness:
    a. Diarrhoea
    b. Cough
    c. Dyspnoea
    d. Myalgia
    e. Fever

30. Transient ischaemic attack:
    a. Symptoms typically last up to 24 hours
    b. Precedes 75% of ischaemic strokes
    c. There may be signs of an ischaemic infarct on brain radiology
    d. CT scan is the preferred radiological investigation
    e. Stroke risk is highest in the first ten days after a TIA

31. Membranous nephropathy:
    a. Secondary membranous nephropathy is more common than primary membranous nephropathy
    b. Is a clinical diagnosis
    c. Spontaneous remission will occur in 90% of those affected
    d. 80% of those with primary membranous nephropathy will have antibodies directed against a specific podocyte antigen
    e. All those affected will have nephrotic syndrome

32. Hypersensitivity pneumonitis:
    a. Requires exposure to particles >5mcg diameter
    b. Is the most common cause of interstitial lung disease
    c. Most commonly occurs due to occupational exposure to industrial chemicals
    d. Will result in a reduced DLCO on lung function testing
    e. Even in the chronic form is reversible once the causative agent is removed

33. Psoriasis:
   a.   Psoriasis vulgaris is the most common type
   b.   Guttate psoriasis will not progress to plaque psoriasis
   c.   Erythrodermic psoriasis will only develop in the plaque psoriasis subtype
   d.   Metabolic syndrome is not more common in those with psoriasis
   e.   Pustular psoriasis is always confined to the hands and feet

34. The size of an aerosol particle transmitted by humans is:
   a.   500-1000µm
   b.   250-500µm
   c.   100-250µm
   d.   5-100µm
   e.   <5µm

35. Which of the following treatments for osteoporosis reduces risk of non vertebral fractures:
   a.   Strontium ranelate
   b.   Oestrogen
   c.   Denusomab
   d.   Selective oestrogen receptor modulators
   e.   Calcitonin

36. Type 1 diabetes:
   a.   Is a monogenic disease
   b.   The majority of those living with type 1 diabetes are under 18 years of age
   c.   Most of those diagnosed with type 1 diabetes have a relative with the disease
   d.   Is associated with complete pancreatic β cell destruction
   e.   50% of cases of cases present in adulthood

37. Hepatitis C virus infection:
    a. Acute infection usually presents with flu-like symptoms
    b. Acute infection usually causes a rise in aminotransferase (ALT) levels more than 10 times the upper limit of normal
    c. Spontaneous clearance of the virus occurs in 90% of those who develop acute hepatitis C infection
    d. Acute hepatitis C infection should be treated with antiviral medication
    e. Those who spontaneously clear hepatitis C infection are not protected from future infection

38. Which of the following is not a risk factor for the development of rheumatoid arthritis:
    a. History of smoking
    b. Breast feeding
    c. Periodontal disease
    d. Older age
    e. Female gender

39. Penicillin allergy:
    a. Anaphylaxis will only occur when penicillin is administered intravenously
    b. Skin prick testing is not useful for diagnosis of IgE mediated penicillin allergy
    c. Genetic testing can be useful to predict immediate penicillin allergic reactions
    d. Desensitisation has been shown to be useful in penicillin allergy
    e. Sensitivity to penicillin allergy does not wane over time

40. Which of the following is not a typical site for scabies rash in adults:
    a. Buttocks
    b. Interdigital spaces of hands
    c. Soles of feet
    d. Face
    e. Genital area

41. Lithium toxicity:

a. Polyuria occurs due to excessive thirst
b. Keeping lithium levels at the lower level of the therapeutic range does not help to reduce polyuria
c. Diuretics are helpful to reduce polyuria
d. Polyuria is the most frequent cause of lithium discontinuation
e. Irreversible renal toxicity does not occur due to lithium treatment

42. Autoinflammatory diseases:

a. Are caused by genetically determined dysfunction of the adaptive immune system
b. Fever episodes should be treated with antibiotics
c. Are characterised by a good therapeutic response to interleukin 8 blockade
d. Are diagnosed by the presence of specific antibodies
e. May overlap with immunodeficiency disorders

43. Natural killer cells:

a. Are neutrophils
b. Are predominantly part of the adaptive immune system
c. Act predominantly against invasive bacteria
d. Develop from CD34$^+$ lymphocytes in the bone marrow
e. Undergo terminal maturation in the bone marrow

44. Which of the following are not more common in individuals with Down syndrome as compared with the general population:

a. Ischaemic heart disease
b. Hypothyroidism
c. Pulmonary hypertension
d. Leukaemia
e. Testicular cancer

45. Transfusion-associated circulatory overload (TACO):

a. Is more common in transfused patients with heart failure than those without heart failure
b. Pulmonary oedema may not be a feature
c. Symptoms must begin within 12 hours of transfusion to fit the definition of TACO
d. BNP levels tend to be higher in transfusion-related acute lung injury (TRALI) as compared with TACO
e. Echocardiography is not useful in distinguishing from TACO from TRALI

46. Chvostek's sign refers to:

a. Contraction of ipsilateral facial muscles after percussion of the facial nerve
b. Contraction of contralateral facial muscles after percussion of the facial nerve
c. Carpopedal spasm after inflation of a sphygmomanometer above the systolic blood pressure
d. Carpopedal spasm after inflation of a sphygmomanometer above the diastolic blood pressure
e. Cortical stress fractures perpendicular to the long axis of the bone

47. Bells palsy:

a. 30% of those with acute peripheral facial palsy will have another cause besides Bell palsy
b. Whether the palsy is partial or complete does not affect the outcome
c. Antiviral treatment reduces the risk of permanent facial palsy
d. Occurs more commonly on the right side of the face
e. The upper facial muscles are spared in Bells palsy

48. The most common inherited thrombophilia is:

a. Prothrombin gene FII G20210A polymorphism
b. Protein C deficiency
c. Protein S deficiency
d. Factor V Leiden
e. Antithrombin deficiency

49. Porphyrias:
a. Can be classified as either renal or erythropoietic
b. Tend to affect the skin or cardiac system
c. Are always autosomal recessive conditions
d. Blistering phototoxicity is a frequent feature
e. Glass can act as an effective barrier to protect against phototoxicity in those with porphyria

50. Paget's disease of bone
a. Is increasing in incidence
b. Can affect the entire skeleton
c. Tends to present under age 50 years
d. Affected sites can transfer to another bone after bone grafting
e. Affected sites may metastasise to other sites spontaneously

51. Rabies:
a. Infection cannot occur through oral ingestion
b. Incubation takes no longer than 14 days
c. Hydrophilia is a clinical feature
d. Tingling around the inoculation site is a common feature
e. Mortality is 40% without treatment

52. Bedbugs:
a. Are almost extinct
b. Their lifecycle comprises six stages
c. May live for years
d. Chemical treatment is essential
e. Require microscopy for diagnosis

53. The most common cause of hyperthyroidism is:
    a.   Toxic nodular goitre
    b.   Graves' disease
    c.   Thyroiditis
    d.   Iodine induced thyroid dysfunction
    e.   Drug induced thyroid dysfunction

54. Diabetic nephropathy:
    a.   All patients with diabetic nephropathy have proteinuria
    b.   Requires the presence of Kimmelstiel-Wilson nodules for diagnosis
    c.   Classification depends mainly on tubulointerstitial renal changes on microscopy
    d.   Hyalinosis of the efferent artericle is a feature by which diabetic nephropathy could be differentiated from hypertensive nephropathy
    e.   Renal lesions associated with type 1 diabetes are more complex than renal lesions associated with type 2 diabetes

55.Physiological aldosterone synthesis is stimulated by:
    a.   Intravascular volume depletion and/or hypokalaemia
    b.   Intravascular volume depletion and/or hyperkalaemia
    c.   Intravascular volume overload and/or hypernatraemia
    d.   Intravascular volume depletion and/or hyponatraemia
    e.   Intravascular volume overload and/or hyperkalaemia

56. Resistant hypertension is defined as:
    a.   Blood pressure >140/90 in spite of treatment with one antihypertensive agent
    b.   Blood pressure >140/90 in spite of treatment with two antihypertensive agents
    c.   Blood pressure >140/90 in spite of treatment with three antihypertensive agents
    d.   Blood pressure >160/90 in spite of treatment with two antihypertensive agents
    e.   Blood pressure >160/90 in spite of treatment with three antihypertensive agents

57. Dexamethasone in COVID-19:
   a. Reduces progression of mild illness
   b. Improves mortality in all patients with COVID-19
   c. Has greatest benefit when started at symptom onset
   d. Reduces mortality in ventilated patients
   e. Does not affect length of hospitalisation

58. The first anti-retroviral used successfully in the treatment of HIV was:
   a. Zidovudine
   b. Tenofovir
   c. Efavirenz
   d. Atazanavir
   e. Lamivudine

59. Cervical spondylosis:
   a. Is more common in women
   b. Is usually associated with neurological symptoms
   c. Less than half of the general population will have cervical disk degeneration on MRI by the age of 50 years
   d. About 10% of people globally will suffer from neck pain
   e. Degenerative changes in the cervical spine may be apparent as early as the first decade of life

60. Chronic lymphocytic leukaemia is a malignancy of:
   a. CD34+ lymphocytes
   b. CD5+ lymphocytes
   c. CD117 lymphocytes
   d. CD45+ lymphocytes
   e. CD8+ lymphocytes

61. Which of the following is more likely to lead to type 2 respiratory failure rather than type 1 respiratory failure:
    a. Opiate toxicity
    b. Pneumonia
    c. Heart failure
    d. Severe COVID-19
    e. Pulmonary embolus

62. Surgical resection for non-small cell lung cancer:
    a. Is potentially curative in all patients
    b. Is potentially curative in stages IA-IVB
    c. Is potentially curative in stages IA-IIIB
    d. Is potentially curative in stages IA-IIB
    e. Is potentially curative in stage I only

63. Pulmonary hypertension is defined as:
    a. Mean pulmonary arterial pressure of 5mmHg or more at rest
    b. Mean pulmonary arterial pressure of 15mmHg or more at rest
    c. Mean pulmonary arterial pressure of 25mmHg or more at rest
    d. Mean pulmonary arterial pressure of 35mmHg or more at rest
    e. Mean pulmonary arterial pressure of 45mmHg or more at rest

64. Which of the following is not one of the Curacao criteria for diagnosis of hereditary haemorrhagic telangiectasia:
    a. Recurrent and spontaneous epistaxis
    b. Visceral localisation
    c. Anaemia due to gastrointestinal bleeding
    d. An affected first degree family member
    e. Mucocutaneous telangiectasia

65. Mesothelioma:
   a.   Always arises from the pleural lining of the lung
   b.   Arises from the peritoneal pleura in 50% of cases
   c.   Involves the pericardium in 20% of cases
   d.   Pleural mesothelioma has become more common than other forms of lung cancer
   e.   Patients with mesothelioma survive on average 12 – 21 months from diagnosis

66. Drug-associated psoriasis:
   a.   Will have a latency period of less than four weeks from exposure to the drugs and onset of psoriasis rash
   b.   Will always resolve on stopping the medication
   c.   May be clinically distinguishable from non-drug associated psoriasis
   d.   May be histologically distinguishable from non-drug associated psoriasis
   e.   Will be refractory to usual topical psoriasis treatments

67. Wilson's disease is caused by mutation in which of the following genes:
   a.   ATP7B
   b.   HFE
   c.   HJP
   d.   SLC40A1
   e.   TFR2

68. Which of the following drugs is least likely to be associated with hyponatraemia:
   a.   Thiazide diuretics
   b.   Loop diuretics
   c.   Lithium
   d.   Fluoxetine
   e.   Venlafaxine

69. Anosmia:

a. Is common in the elderly
b. Occurs in 90% of those with COVID-19
c. Is usually permanent when caused by COVID-19
d. COVID-19 may affect smell but not taste
e. Requires investigation even when transient

70. Bacillus Calmette-Guerin (BCG) vaccination:

a. Is a live attenuated form of Mycobacterium tuberculosis
b. Is used in the treatment of invasive bladder cancer
c. May cause disseminated BCG infection
d. All children worldwide should receive the vaccination
e. Protects only against Mycobacterium tuberculosis

71. The most common bacterial cause of native valve endocarditis is:

a. Streptococcus viridans
b. Coagulase negative staphyloccccus
c. Staphylococcus aureus
d. Streptococcus gallolyticus
e. Haemophilus influenza

72. Which of the following are not included in the diagnostic criteria for polymyalgia rheumatica:

a. Morning stiffness
b. Hip pain
c. Absence of rheumatoid factor or anti-citrullinated protein antibody
d. Subdeltoid bursitis
e. Temporal headache

73. Postural tachycardia syndrome (POTS):

a.   Is associated with increased mortality
b.   Requires demonstration of postural hypotension for diagnosis
c.   Requires tilt table testing for diagnosis
d.   Requires a history of syncope for diagnosis
e.   Requires a demonstration of postural tachycardia for diagnosis

74. Joint hypermobility:

a.   Is always generalised
b.   Always leads to pain symptoms
c.   Is linked to a specific genetic cause
d.   Is diagnosed using the Villefranche criteria
e.   Has overlap with heritable connective tissue disorders

75. Trigeminal neuralgia:

a.   May cause continuous pain
b.   Requires an MRI scan for diagnosis
c.   Is often bilateral
d.   Most of those affected do not have triggered pain
e.   Most commonly affects the first branch of the trigeminal nerve

76. The most common symptoms seen in post-acute COVID-19 are:

a.   Cough, low grade fever and fatigue
b.   Palpitations, lightheadedness and shortness of breath
c.   Headaches, chest pain and fatigue
d.   Visual disturbance, loss of taste and loss of smell
e.   Chronic pain, arthralgia and myalgia

77. Congenital colour vision deficiency:
    a.   Affects blue-yellow colour perception most commonly
    b.   Occurs due to genetic abnormalities leading to abnormal function of rod photoreceptors
    c.   Is more common in Africans than Europeans
    d.   Is usually autosomal dominant
    e.   Is more common in males than females

78. Thyroid nodules:
    a.   Are present in about 10% of people at autopsy
    b.   50% of radiologically detected nodules are malignant
    c.   Are more common in men
    d.   CT scan is the best radiological modality for assessment of thyroid nodules
    e.   Microcalcifications on ultrasound suggests a malignant nodule

79. Carbon monoxide poisoning:
    a.   Smokers are more vulnerable to carbon monoxide toxicity than non-smokers
    b.   Cherry red skin tone is pathognomonic
    c.   Oxygen saturation measured by pulse oximetry is reliable in diagnosis
    d.   Carboxyhaemoglobin levels of 15-20% will cause toxic effects
    e.   Patients should not be given 100% oxygen

80. Which of the following is not associated with increased risk of developing primary biliary cirrhosis (PBC):
    a.   Tobacco smoking
    b.   Excessive alcohol intake
    c.   Recurrent urinary tract infections
    d.   Female gender
    e.   Positive family history of PBC

81. In 1964 a 16-month old girl with normal hearing was noted to have recurring episodes of collapse, assumed to be psychogenic. At the age of 6 she was investigated again for an organic cause. She was noted to have a prolonged QT interval on ECG. While playing on the ward she collapsed in ventricular fibrillation. She recovered and her symptoms improved with betablocker treatment. A brother also had prolonged QT interval and frequent syncopes and died in childhood. What is the diagnosis:
   a.   Wolf Parkinson White syndrome
   b.   Jervell Lange Nielson syndrome
   c.   Romano Ward syndrome
   d.   Brugada syndrome
   e.   Arrhythmogenic right ventricular cardiomyopathy

82. Pregabalin most has proven efficacy in:
   a.   Nociceptive pain
   b.   Sciatica
   c.   Neuropathic pain
   d.   Post-operative pain
   e.   Migraine

83. Generic medications:
   a.   Should not be used interchangeably with branded medications
   b.   When studied generic cardiovascular medications were found to have no significant difference to originator medications
   c.   Are shown to be of inferior efficacy to branded medications
   d.   Are more likely to cause adverse effects than branded medications
   e.   Generic anticonvulsants should not be used

84. Which of the following antibiotics has the least risk of causing Clostridioides difficile infection:
   a.   Vancomycin
   b.   Amoxicillin
   c.   Ceftriaxone
   d.   Ciprofloxacin
   e.   Clindamycin

85. Which of the following is <u>not</u> a known side effect of cholinesterase inhibitors used for the treatment of dementia:
    a. Muscle cramps
    b. Nausea
    c. Vivid dreams
    d. Tachycardia
    e. Insomnia

86. Which of the following is <u>not</u> a risk factor for bleeding on anticoagulation:
    a. Uncontrolled hypertension with systolic blood pressure >160mmHg
    b. Severe renal disease
    c. Dementia
    d. Associated use of low dose aspirin
    e. Labile INR on warfarin

87. Herpes zoster ophthalmicus:
    a. Occurs due to varicella zoster virus recurrence involving the facial nerve
    b. Optic neuritis is the most common complication
    c. Will not affect the retina
    d. Glaucoma may occur
    e. Hutchinson sign refers to rash affecting the orbit indicating ocular involvement

88. The most common form of dementia occurring in those under the age of 65 years is:
    a. Alzheimer's dementia
    b. Lewy body dementia
    c. Frontotemporal dementia
    d. Vascular dementia
    e. Jakob Creutzfeldt disease

89. Autoantibodies that target components of hemidesmosomes in the basement membrane zone lead to blistering in:
   a. Pemphigus
   b. Pemphigoid
   c. Allergic contact dermatitis
   d. Dermatitis herpetiformis
   e. Herpes zoster

90. 90% of drug induced autoimmune hepatitis is caused by:
   a. Methyldopa and diclofenac
   b. Atorvastatin and liraglutide
   c. Herbal medications
   d. Nitrofurantoin and minocycline
   e. Interferon α and interferon σ

91. Familial hypercholesterolaemia is primarily a disorder of:
   a. Triglycerides
   b. HDL
   c. LDL
   d. VLDL
   e. Total cholesterol

92. Dix Hallpike manoeuvre:
   a. Nystagmus should begin immediately on lying flat in a positive test
   b. Nystagmus will not occur after sitting upright after a positive test
   c. Nystagmus will persist for a similar time period with repeated testing
   d. Intensity of nystagmus correlates with severity of vertigo
   e. Hanging the head over the back if the bed on lying flat is necessary when performing Dix-Hallpike manoeuvre

93. Anti RNA polymerase III antibody positivity is associated with:
    a. Undifferentiated connective tissue disorder
    b. Mixed connective tissue disorder
    c. Morphoea
    d. CREST syndrome
    e. Diffuse cutaneous systemic scleroderma

94. Which of the following is not a typical feature of Guillain Barre syndrome:
    a. Progressive weakness
    b. Brisk tendon reflexes
    c. Raised cerebrospinal fluid protein levels
    d. Maximal weakness reached within four weeks of onset
    e. Blood pressure instability

95. Polycystic kidney disease:
    a. Is a cilia-related disorder
    b. Autosomal recessive polycystic kidney disease is more common than autosomal dominant polycystic kidney disease
    c. Autosomal recessive polycystic kidney disease has a less severe course than autosomal dominant polycystic kidney disease
    d. Autosomal recessive polycystic kidney disease tends to present later than autosomal dominant polycystic kidney disease
    e. Autosomal recessive polycystic kidney disease and autosomal dominant polycystic kidney disease rarely progress to end-stage renal disease

96. C-peptide:
    a. Levels are affected by exogenous insulin use
    b. Is undetectable in type 1 diabetes
    c. Is undetectable in type 2 diabetes
    d. Is the investigation of choice where diagnostic uncertainty exists between a diagnosis of type 1 and type 2 diabetes
    e. Is a by-product of insulin release

97. Interferon-γ-release assays:

    a.   Are used primarily to diagnose active tuberculosis infection

    b.   Can distinguish between active and latent tuberculosis infection

    c.   Will not cross-react with non-tuberculous mycobacteria

    d.   Will not cross-react with BCG vaccination

    e.   Detect B-cell antibodies to tuberculosis

98. Hepatorenal syndrome:

    a.   Serum creatinine overestimates renal function deterioration in patient with liver cirrhosis

    b.   Urine output is a more useful guide to acute kidney injury than serum creatinine in those with cirrhosis

    c.   Renal damage is irreversible in hepatorenal syndrome

    d.   Severity of ascites is a risk factor for hepatorenal syndrome development

    e.   Occurs due to structural kidney injury secondary to pre-renal azotaemia from hypovolaemia

99. Gout:

    a.   Most people with hyperuricaemia will develop gout

    b.   Is more common in men than women only over the age of 60 years

    c.   Starting at lower doses of uric acid lowering treatment does not reduce risk of acute gout flares

    d.   Immunosuppressed organ transplant recipients can progress to chronic tophaceous gout within 3 to 5 years

    e.   Rheumatoid arthritis is the main differential diagnosis at presentation

100. The drugs which most commonly cause idiosyncratic drug-induced liver injury worldwide are:

    a.   Antiepileptic drugs

    b.   Antimicrobial drugs

    c.   Antihypertensive drugs

    d.   Statins

    e.   Immunomodulators

1. Answer c

Dyspnoea is the most common symptom in aortic stenosis with exertional angina, pre-syncope and syncope occurring in more severe disease. Sudden cardiac death is also a risk.[6]

2. Answer b

Food-bound cobalamin malabsorption (FBCM) is the most common cause of vitamin B12 deficiency. It is caused by failure of cobalamin or vitamin B12 to dissociate from food proteins, often due to reduced stomach acidity. Proton pump inhibitor use is one of the possible causes, and metformin has also been associated with reduced vitamin B12 levels. Although intramuscular vitamin B12 replacement has traditionally been thought necessary, there is increasing evidence that oral replacement may be sufficient. The manifestations of vitamin B12 deficiency due to FBCM tends to be less severe than those due to pernicious anaemia but neurological manifestations may still occur.[9]

3. Answer a

4. Answer c

Acute urticaria is urticarial rash lasting less than 6 weeks. It may be triggered by medications, foods or other exposures. Urticaria arising from pressure is known as inducible urticaria and is a form of chronic urticaria. In 50% of cases there is no clear trigger and this is known as acute spontaneous urticaria. The rash resolves spontaneous y and will not scar. Any known triggers should be avoided as exposure may lead to anaphylaxis.[16]

5. Answer a

Light microscopy of Giemsa-stained blood film is the gold standard for diagnosis of malaria. It may need to be repeated at 12 and 24 hours if initially negative in case of low level parasitaemia. It is operator dependent and requires some expertise, and not always available in endemic areas.

Rapid diagnostic testing for antigens is becoming increasingly sensitive and is recommended in endemic areas as an initial screening test by the World Health Organisation, but positive results should be confirmed with blood smears. Polymerase chain reaction is useful for low level parasitaemia and serology testing for antibodies such as ELISA can also be performed.[21,22,23]

6. Answer e

Alpha-1 antitrypsin deficiency is inherited in an autosomal recessive manner. The Pi*MM genotype indicates non-affected individuals. The Pi*ZZ term is used to indicate a homozygote and Pi*MZ indicates a heterozygote. Some non-smokers may not develop lung disease. It may manifest as liver cirrhosis in children and even neonates. Alpha-1 antitrypsin may act as an acute phase reactant but levels in homozygotes should still be below the normal range.[24]

7. Answer c

Cataract is the most common cause of blindness worldwide, causing 51% of world blindness. Its incidence is expected to grow as the world population ages.

Trachoma has been the leading infectious cause of blindness. It is caused by chlamydia trachomatis, and is endemic in many developing countries. It causes a scarring infection of eyelids and leads to entropion and trichiasis with resulting corneal scarring. It's eradication has been prioritised by the WHO through the SAFE programme (Surgery to treat blinding disease, antibiotics to clear infection, facial cleanliness and environmental improvement) which has greatly reduced its prevalence.[23,35, 36]

8. Answer b

Although smoking cessation is the most beneficial intervention with regard to improving the natural history of COPD, the disease is a progressive one in all patients. The GOLD guidelines classify COPD according to lung function, patient-reported symptoms and exacerbations and recommends stepwise treatments depending on this classification. Long term use of macrolide antibiotics has been shown to reduce exacerbations by 27% but does not alter disease progression. Inhaled corticosteroids as monotherapy are not recommended in COPD due to increased risk of pneumonia. However inhaled corticosteroids are included in GOLD stepwise treatment recommendations as part of 'triple therapy' with an inhaled long-acting beta-agonist and an inhaled long-acting muscarinic antagonist for those with high symptom burden and frequent exacerbations. The benefits of pulmonary rehabilitation have been shown to exceed those of pharmacological management, including benefits in symptom control and quality of life.[53]

9. Answer d

Natriuretic peptides (brain natriuretic peptide or BNP and N-terminal pro BNP or NT-proBNP) are proteins which increase in heart failure. Obesity causes a decrease in natriuretic peptides while all the others listed are non-cardiac causes of a rise in natriuretic peptides.[56,57,58]

10. Answer b

Primary adrenal insufficiency (PAI) is also known as Addison's disease. 80% of PAI is autoimmune. Long term steroid therapy causes secondary adrenal insufficiency. Oral hydrocortisone is the replacement treatment of choice, followed by oral prednisolone. Oral dexamethasone is unsuitable as it has a long half-life which is atypical of endogenous steroids. Oral steroid should be given twice daily with the higher dose in the morning to mimic physiological diurnal variation. Replacement therapy can be monitored clinically as monitoring ACTH or cortisol levels are not useful. Dynamic testing with Synacthen test may be needed for diagnosis. [73]

11. Answer a

Primary mitral regurgitation (MR) occurs due to a primary mitral valvular problem, as opposed to secondary mitral regurgitation which occurs due to disease of the atrium or ventricle. It may be asymptomatic and mild with compensation by run-off into the left atrium. However it may progress to more severe decompensated MR with symptoms and left ventricular dysfunction. Natural history studies have shown a 90% mortality over 10 years for primary MR, with 63% incidence of heart failure and 30%

incidence of atrial fibrillation. The outcome of patients with MR is related to symptoms at presentation (mortality increases from NYHA I to IV) and the level of left ventricular dysfunction. Once symptoms develop ventricular dysfunction is irreversible with a poor prognosis so earlier operative intervention is preferred. Advances in operative management have improved outcomes and mitral valve repair is associated with lower mortality and fewer complications than mitral valve replacement.

The direction of radiation of the murmur can help identify the valvular leaflet involved. Radiation to the left sternal border may indicate posterior leaflet involvement, while a posterior directed murmur indicates anterior leaflet involvement.[77]

12. Answer d

PCR is the most common method for detecting respiratory viruses at present.[78]

13. Answer a

80% of those with SJS/TEN have mucosal involvement with oral involvement the most common.[92]

14. Answer a

Methotrexate adverse effects include nausea, headaches, fatigue, hair loss, mucositis, liver fibrosis and cirrhosis, interstitial pneumonitis and cytopenias. The most common are gastrointestinal (nausea, vomiting, stomatitis and hepatotoxicity).[98]

15. Answer d

Pectus excavatum is a dorsal displacement of the sternum and constitutes 90% of all chest wall deformities. Most defects are apparent within the first year or life, with 80% apparent by age 2. It affects males 5 times more than females. There is an associated connective tissue disease in < 1% of cases. There are many associated conditions including Marfan syndrome, Noonan syndrome, primary ciliary dyskinesia and osteogenesis imperfecta, as well as an association with cardiac abnormalities. Although often asymptomatic

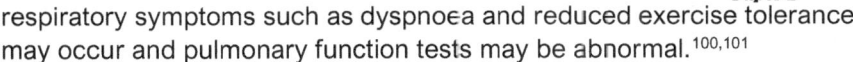

respiratory symptoms such as dyspnoea and reduced exercise tolerance may occur and pulmonary function tests may be abnormal.[100,101]

16. Answer a

Valvular atrial fibrillation refers to atrial fibrillation associated with rheumatic mitral stenosis or mechanical prosthetic valve. Stroke risk is increased in this group compared with those with non-valvular atrial fibrillation, and thrombus is less likely to come from the left atrium for reasons unknown. Vitamin K antagonists such as warfarin are preferab e to direct oral anti coagulants at present in valvular atrial fibrillation. This is mainly due to the RE-ALIGN trial which showed that dabigatran was inferior to warfarin for stroke prevention in valvular atrial fibrillation with moderate to severe dysfunction. The European Heart Association classify patients with atrial fibrillation and valvular abnormalities into two groups. EHRA (Evaluated Heart valves, Rheumatic or Artificial) type 1 is valvular atrial fibrillation with mitral stenosis or mechanical prosthetic valve. EHRA type 2 which is atrial fibrillation associated with other valve disorders such as aortic stenosis or regurgitation or mitral regurgitation where vitamin K antagonists or direct oral anti coagulants may be used for stroke prevention.[102]

17. Answer a

Anti-transglutaminase (tTG) antibodies and anti-endomysium (EmA) antibodies are both IgA antibodies. Anti-tTG antibodies are more sensitive but less specific that EmA antibodies (anti-tTG antibodies are 97% sensitive and 91% specific and EmA antibodies are 94% sensitive and 100% specific). DGP antibodies are IgG antibodies that are less useful in adults but can be useful in diagnosing coeliac disease in younger children. Antibodies in most individuals will reduced significantly or return to normal within 12 to 24 months with strict compliance with a gluten free diet, but this does not necessarily reflect regrowth of intestinal villi.[105]

18. Answer d

Acromegaly is caused by growth-hormone secret ng somatotroph pituitary tumours. It is usually insidious presenting due to concerns over changes in appearance, dental or orthopaedic problems or secondary cardiovascular respiratory or cerebrovascular effects. 70% are caused by an invasive adenoma. Growth hormone secretion is highly pulsatile and static testing is not useful for diagnosis. Elevated IGF1 (insulin-like growth factor-1) levels are specific but dynamic testing with a glucose tolerance test is required for diagnosis, showing a high nadir of growth hormone levels after a 75g glucose challenge. Obstructive sleep apnoea is a common association in untreated acromegaly. Dopamine agonist treatment is used in mild disease.[109]

19. Answer d

Helicobacter pylori is a gram-negative bacterium thought to be present in humans for thousands of years. It is associated with benign and malignant gastrointestinal conditions. It has some unusual properties in that it can survive in an acidic environment, and unusually for a gram negative organism it is sensitive to penicillin. Given its association with insidious gastrointestinal conditions such as chronic active gastritis and gastric neoplasms it is eradicated with antibiotic treatment when detected, unless there are competing considerations. It has been classified as a group 1 carcinogen (strong evidence for an association with cancer) by the International Agency for Research on Cancer, a World Health Organisation body.[115,116,117]

20. Answer e

Pityriasis rosea is a self-limiting rash thought to be triggered by systemic reactivation of human herpesvirus (HHV) 6 and/or HHV 7. It begins with an erythematous scaly herald patch which may be present for two weeks prior to onset of a more generalised rash consisting of smaller scaly papulosquamous lesions mainly on the trunk. It may relapse within one year in 2-3% of patients, usually without a herald patch and tends to be shorter and less widespread than the initial episode. Persistent pityriasis rosea lasts longer than 12 weeks and is usually associated with systemic symptoms. It is reported to be more common in pregnancy than in the general population (18% vs 6%), possibly due to an altered immune response, and if occurring within the 15th week of gestation is associated with increased risk of miscarriage.[120]

21. Answer d

Exacerbations in chronic obstructive pulmonary disease are shown to accelerate progression of the disease, affect underlying health status and increase mortality. The frequency and severity of exacerbations is associated with long-term mortality independent of comorbidities, FEV1, age and body mass index. Long term azithromycin has been shown to reduce exacerbations (hazard ratio 0.74) although it is uncertain if this is due to an anti-bacterial or immunomodulatory effect.[123]

22. Answer d

Flecainide is a Vaughn-Williams Class IC agent. It has a negative inotropic effect and it is contraindicated in those with reduced ejection fraction or heart failure. It may prolong the PR interval or QRS complex on a 12-lead ECG but does not lead to prolonged QT interval or increase torsade de pointes risk. Placebo-controlled trials have shown its efficacy in conversion of acute atrial fibrillation to sinus rhythm and also in maintenance of sinus rhythm in those with a history of atrial fibrillation. In the 1980s the CAST study, which was designed to assess whether a range of anti-arrhythmics could reduce sudden death in patients with frequent ventricular ectopics and reduced ejection fraction following a recent MI, showed increased mortality for flecainide. This has led to concerns about its pro-arrhythmic effects in those with a structurally abnormal heart. However its safety in a structurally normal heart is well established.[124]

23. Answer a

Lymphopenia rather than lymphocytosis is a typical feature of COVID 19.[125]

24. Answer d

Hodgkin's lymphoma is a malignancy arising from germinal centre and post-germinal centre B cells. It is characterised by the presence of multinucleate giant cells or large mononuclear cells known as Hodgkin and Reed Sternberg (HRS) cells. Malignant cells make up the minority of the tumours with a background infiltrate of inflammatory cells. It accounts for 10% of all lymphomas. There is an association with Epstein Barr virus although this appears to be strongest in the developing world and in those with HIV, and it is found in Hodgkin's lymphoma much less frequently in the industrialised world. Immunosuppression is a risk factor, with increased risk in HIV infection, solid organ transplantation, rheumatoid arthritis and systemic lupus erythematosus.[129,130]

25. Answer a

The most common areas affected in Crohn's disease are the ileum and colon, affecting 37%. Colon only affects 35%. Small bowel only affects 28% and gastroduodenal area affects 5%.[131]

26. Answer a

Amiodarone is a class III antiarrhythmic. 90% of those on amiodarone will remain euthyroid. A 200mg amiodarone tablet contains 500 times the recommended daily allowance of iodine. The effects of amiodarone on the thyroid are related to its high iodine content and also its direct toxic effect on thyroid parenchyma. It is more likely to cause hypothyroidism in thyroid-sufficient areas. This can be triggered in those with or without existing anti-thyroid antibodies and is more common in women. It is less likely to resolve after stopping amiodarone in those with pre-existing thyroid autoimmunity and lifelong replacement thyroid hormone may be needed.

Amiodarone induced thyrotoxicosis is more likely to occur in thyroid-deficient areas. It may be an unmasking of an underlying toxic multinodular goitre or Grave's disease, or it may occur due to a toxic thyroiditis releasing pre-formed thyroid hormone. A combination of both may occur. Treatment may involve corticosteroid use in thyroiditis, or antithyroid medications. Due to the long half-life of amiodarone thyroid abnormalities may persist for months after stopping the medications.[134]

27. Answer a

Primary immunodeficiencies are a group of heterogeneous disorders characterised by immune system abnormalities with various combinations of recurring infections, lymphoproliferation, granulomatous processes, autoimmunity, atopy, and malignancy. The most common type is common variable immunodeficiency which is characterised by hypogammaglobulinemia and recurrent infections.[171,174]

28. Answer a

The most common presenting symptom in ulcerative colitis is rectal bleeding.[142]

29. Answer c

The most common presenting symptoms of COVID 19 are fever, cough, fatigue, anorexia, myalgias and diarrhoea. Dyspnoea is the most common sign of progression to severe disease which usually develops after one week of illness.[149]

30. Answer e

Transient ischaemic attack (TIA) involves transient neurological signs or symptoms usually lasting seconds to minutes and usually less than one hour, with no radiological signs of an acute ischaemc infarct on brain radiology. The previous definition of symptoms lasting less than 24 hours has been revised due to the finding that events lasting as little as 10 minutes may cause detectable ischaemia on radiological investigations such as MRI, and urgent revascularisation may be attempted within 6 hours of onset of symptoms. The presence of an infarct on brain imaging results in a diagnosis of a minor stroke rather than TIA. 20-25% of stroke events are preceded by transient ischaemic symptoms. Without intervention the risk of stroke is as high as 20% after a TIA, with most of the risk in the first 10 days after the event. Diffusion weighted imaging assessed with MRI scan is the radiological test of choice for investigation to exclude an acute ischaemic event.[150]

31. Answer d

Membranous nephropathy is the most common cause of nephrotic syndrome in white adults. It usually presents with severe proteinuria, oedema, hypoalbuminaemia and hyperlipidaemia. It requires renal biopsy for diagnosis, with characteristic histopathological features of subepithelial immune complex deposits and subsequent glomerular basement membrane thickening. About 20% of cases are secondary to other conditions, such as autoimmune conditions (SLE, rheumatoid arthritis), infection (hepatitis B and C) malignancy (colon or lung cancer) and drugs (gold, penicillamine). Spontaneous remission occurs in 30%, usually within the first two years of diagnosis. Primary membranous nephropathy is associated with antibodies against specific podocyte antigens, in particular M-type phospholipase A2 receptor (PLA$_2$R). 80% of those with membranous nephropathy will develop nephrotic syndrome.[154,155]

32. Answer d

Hypersensitivity pneumonitis is a delayed allergic reaction to external agents leading to inflammation of the alveoli, terminal bronchioles and alveolar interstitium. It most commonly occurs due to exposure to organic animal or vegetable dusts, with chemical causes much less common. It causes only a small proportion of interstitial lung disease, with other causes such as idiopathic pulmonary fibrosis and lung fibrosis secondary to underlying connective tissue disease more common. It requires exposure to particles sufficiently small to reach the alveoli (<5mcg diameter). It can present acutely with cough, fever and dyspnoea, or as chronic disease, with progressive pulmonary fibrosis which is not reversible. Pulmonary function testing usually shows a restrictive pattern although there may be obstructive features, and DLCO is reduced.[156,157]

33. Answer a

Psoriasis subtypes include plaque-type psoriasis (psoriasis vulgaris), inverse psoriasis, guttate psoriasis and pustular psoriasis. Plaque type psoriasis is the most common, constituting 90% of cases. Guttate psoriasis is an acute form with small erythematous plaques, often triggered by group A streptococcal tonsillitis. One third will progress to plaque psoriasis. Any type of psoriasis can progress to erythrodermic psoriasis, where over 90% of body surface area is affected. Increased BMI, hypertension, cardiovascular disease, type 2 diabetes and hyperlipidaemia all occur more frequently in those with psoriasis and the metabolic syndrome is twice as frequent in those with psoriasis as compared with the general population. Pustular psoriasis may predominantly affect the hands and feet, or may develop an acute progressive course with generalised rash and systemic symptoms.[158]

34. Answer e

Human respiratory droplets are exhaled during breathing, speaking, coughing and sneezing. They can range in size from 0.1 to 1000μm. Smaller aerosols (<5μm) are less likely to settle and can be transmitted by air currents for significant distances.[159]

35. Answer c

Most of the listed treatments have fallen out of favour for the treatment of osteoporosis for various reasons. The treatments with known benefits for reducing both vertebral and non vertebral fracture risk are denusomab (a human monoclonal antibody to the receptor activator of NF - alpha B ligand), bisphosphonates (analogues of pyrophosphate compounds) and teriparatide (a truncated form of parathyroid hormore). These three medications currently form the basis for osteoporosis treatment and fracture prevention.[160]

36. Answer e

Type 1 diabetes is a polygenic disease, with its pathogenesis not completely understood. Although often presenting in childhood, the peak incidence is in children aged 10-14 years of age. 50% of cases present in adulthood and most of those living with type 1 diabetes are adults. Although it is a heritable polygenic disease with identical twin concordance of 30-70%, most of those diagnosed do not have a relative with the disease. There is usually significant pancreatic β cell reserve at diagnosis and although this wanes with time, there is still evidence of some β cell function in many of those with long standing type 1 diabetes.[161]

37. Answer e

Acute hepatitis C virus (HCV) infection is usually asymptomatic although there may be flu-like symptoms or jaundice. High rises of aminotransferases about 10 times the upper limit of normal are unusual in acute infection. 15-25%% of those with acute infection will clear the virus. In acute infection, deferral of treatment is recommended for 6 months to see if the virus will spontaneously clear. In practice however it is often difficult to distinguish acute from chronic infection. Persistence of HCV antibodies in those who clear acute HCV infection does not protect against future infection.[162,163]

38. Answer b

Breast feeding decreases the risk of developing rheumatoid arthritis, while early menarche and very irregular menses increases risk.

Current and previous smoking with relative risk up to 2.2 for a 40 pack year history of smoking. Older age, female gender, obesity and positive family history are also known risk factors.

Periodontal disease can increase risk, with studies showing that infection with the common periodontal bacterium Porphyromonas gingivalis can result in the induction of autoimmune response by the citrullination of host peptides.[164,165]

39. Answer d

Penicillin allergy may consist of immediate IgE mediated reactions such as urticaria or anaphylaxis, exanthemum type skin rashes or delayed reactions such as DRESS or SJS-TEN reactions. Anaphylaxis may occur following oral, intravenous or subcutaneous administration. Skin prick testing is useful in diagnosis of IgE mediated penicillin allergy. Although an association between HLA typing and some delayed reactions in penicillin allergy have been found, genetic testing is not useful in predicting penicillin allergy in general. Skin prick testing ten years following a known penicillin reaction has shown that allergy may wane over time. Desensitisation by exposure to incrementally increasing doses of penicillin has been used in individuals with IgE mediated penicillin allergy where penicillin is seen as essential and has been shown to be effective.[166]

40. Answer d

Scabies is an infestation caused by the female scabies mite Sarcoptes scabiei. It is generally benign but highly transmissible. Typical areas of distribution in adults are the interdigital web space of the fingers, wrists, inner elbows, the soles of the feet, around the breasts and axillae, scrotal and penile areas and on the buttocks, knees and shoulder blades.[167,168]

41. Answer c

Polyuria and polydipsia are common adverse effects to lithium treatment occurring in up to 70% of those treated. It is usually well tolerated and other adverse effects are more likely to lead to discontinuation. Lithium interferes with the renal collecting tubules reducing the retention of free water, and so polyuria leads to thirst and polydipsia. Keeping lithium levels low can help to minimise this side effect. Paradoxically diuretics such as amiloride and hydrochlorothiazide have been shown to be effective in reducing polyuria. About 20% of those on long term lithium treatment will develop irreversible renal damage although how polyuria reflects this renal toxicity is uncertain.[169]

42. Answer e

Autoinflammatory diseases are characterised by repeated episodes of sterile inflammation, with periodic fevers and a variety of other features such as skin rashes, arthralgias, myalgias and serositis to name a few. Fever episodes tend to resolve spontaneously. They are caused by a genetically determined dysfunction of the innate immune system without development of autoantibodies or autoreactive T cells. In spite of the fact that they are a heterogenous group of disorders caused by a variety of genetic mutations, they tend to respond to interleukin 1 (IL1) blockade with anakinra (recombinant anti-IL1 receptor antagonist) and canakinumab (anti-IL1β monoclonal antibody). Overlap is seen with primary immunodeficiency disorders with some common features.[173]

43. Answer d

Natural killer cells are lymphocytes and are predominantly part of the innate immune system. They act mainly against viruses. Other roles for NK cells have been discovered in recent years including immunoregulatory functions and effects on the adaptive immune system. They develop from $CD34^+$ lymphocytes in the bone marrow and they undergo terminal maturation in the peripheral lymphoid tissue.[170]

44. Answer a

Down syndrome or trisomy 21 is associated with increased risk of many conditions as compared with the general population.

Pulmonary hypertension with or without congenital heart disease is more common, as well as obesity, gastro oesophageal reflux and obstructive sleep apnoea.

Haematological abnormalities are more common, including a transient abnormal myelopoiesis, a form of myeloid preleukaemia which progresses to leukaemia in 20 to 30% of cases. The overall risk of leukaemia independent of transient abnormal myelopoiesis is 2 to 3 % of all individuals with Down syndrome.

Down syndrome appears to be protective against most solid tumours although testicular cancer is more common in age-matched individuals.

Autoimmune conditions in general are more common including Hashimoto's disease, type 1 diabetes, alopecia and coeliac disease. The incidence of thyroid abnormalities is approximately 50% by age 45 in those with Down syndrome. All individuals with Down syndrome should have annual thyroid function testing.

Ischaemic heart disease may occur in adults with Down syndrome but is less common than in the general population.[175]

45. Answer a

Transfusion-associated circulatory overload (TACO) and transfusion-related acute lung injury (TRALI) are potentially fatal transfusion reactions. Acute pulmonary oedema within 6 hours of completion of blood product transfusion is common to both conditions. TACO is defined as acute pulmonary oedema within 6 hours of transfusion with evidence of circulatory overload (three or more of acute respiratory distress, radiographic pulmonary oedema, elevated central venous pressure, evidence of left heart failure, elevated BNP, positive fluid balance). Risk is higher in those with heart failure or renal impairment where there may be impaired mechanisms to compensate for an increase in circulating blood values. TRALI is acute pulmonary oedema within 6 hours of completing transfusion without signs of circulatory overload or other ARDS risk factor. BNP tends to be elevated in TACO and not TRALI. Echocardiographic findings can also help to distinguish the two conditions.[176]

46. Answer a

Chvostek's sign refers to contraction of ipsilateral facial muscles after percussion of the facial nerve seen in hypocalcaemia.

Carpopedal spasm after inflation of a sphygmomanometer above the systolic blood pressure is known as Trousseau's signs, also seen in hypocalcaemia.

Cortical stress fractures perpendicular to the long axis of the bone are known as Looser zones and are classic radiographic findings of osteomalacia.[177]

47. Answer a

Bells palsy is an acute lower motor neurone facial palsy. Those with complete paralysis are less likely to have a full recovery than those with partial paralysis (paresis). Up to 30% of acute lower motor neurone facial palsy will have another cause which is not Bells palsy. Acute suppurative ear disease, Ramsay Hunt syndrome, parotid tumour and Lyme disease are potential differentials. Corticosteroid treatment reduces the risk of permanent facial weakness, but antiviral treatment has not been shown to affect outcome. It may occur on either side of the face with equal frequency. Upper facial muscle sparing suggests an upper motor neurone weakness and an alternative diagnosis.[178]

48. Answer d

Factor V Leiden is the most common inherited thrombophilia followed by prothrombin gene FII G20210A polymorphism (PGM). Deficiencies in protein C, protein S and antithrombin are less common inherited thrombophilias.[179]

49. Answer d

Porphyrias consist of nine conditions characterised by alterations in enzymes involved in heme biosynthesis. There is overproduction of heme precursors in either the liver or bone marrow, leading to a classification of porphyrias as either hepatic or erythropoietic. The major clinical manifestations are either cutaneous from phototoxicity, or neurological. The conditions may be autosomal dominant with variable penetrance, autosomal recessive or X linked. Blistering phototoxicity can be a feature. The light that maximally photoactivates porphyrias passes through glass so it is not an effective barrier in porphyrias.[181]

50. Answer d

Paget's disease of bone is a disorder of bone turnover, characterised by abnormalities in osteoclast and osteoblast function leading to foci of disordered bone formation. It has been most prominent in populations of English descent and is decreasing rapidly in incidence, so that is it now an uncommon condition. There is thought to be a genetic predisposition with triggering environmental factors. Viral infection is thought to play a role but this has never been proven. It affects various sites and can affect any bone, but never the entire skeleton. It is rare under the age of 50 years and incidence increases in the elderly. Affected sites will not migrate to other bones spontaneously but transference to another bone has been described after bone grafting.[182,183]

51. Answer d

Rabies is a viral infection caused by a virus of the rhabdoviridae family of viruses. It is usually transmitted via a bite or scratch from an infected mammal, via saliva. It may be transmitted via ingestion, transplacentally or even through organ transplants. The incubation period following inoculation can take from two weeks to six years, so an animal bite may not be remembered. Tingling at the bite site is a consistent feature. Clinical course involves a prodrome of fever, malaise and headache followed by agitation and confusion, progressing to paralysis and death. Frothing at the mouth occurs due to hypersalivation. There may be intense pharyngeal spasm at the sight or sound of water, known as hydrophobia. The disease is uniformly fatal without treatment.[184,185,186]

52. Answer b

Bedbugs are Cimex lectularis (common bedbug) and Cimex hemipterus (tropical bed bugs) They are resurgent around the world for many reasons, including resistance to chemical treatments and increases in international travel (until recently). Their lifecycle comprises six stages: egg, four lymphal stages and adult. They may survive up to 4 to 5 months if they have a food source. They cause insect bites although these cannot be differentiated from insect bites from other sources. Hotels, hospitals and cruise ships are particularly vulnerable to outbreaks but they may occur anywhere. Exoskeletons and faeces can be seen with the naked eye They tend to hide in dark crevices and come out at night for a blood meal from a sleeping host. Non chemical management is essential, such as washing bed clothes at 60°C and hoovering. Chemical treatments are likely to be less useful due to resistance.[187]

53. Answer b

Hyperthyroidism is a state of increased production and secretion of thyroid hormone from the thyroid gland. Thyrotoxicosis is a clinical syndrome of excess circulating thyroid hormone of any cause. Graves' disease is the most common cause of hyperthyroidism, at least in iodine sufficient areas. Toxic nodular goitre is the second most common cause. Thyroiditis, iodine induced and drug induced thyroid dysfunction, as well as excess intake of thyroid hormone, are causes of thyrotoxicosis.[188]

54. Answer d

Diabetic nephropathy is one of the major causes of end-stage renal failure worldwide. It is characterised primarily by pathological glomerular lesions. These manifest initially as diffuse and nodular mesangial expansion and glomerular basement membrane thickening. These lesions develop within 2 to 8 years after diagnosis of diabetes mellitus. Diffuse mesangial expansion progresses to nodular accumulation of mesangial matrix, known as Kimmelsteil Wilson nodules. These are present in about 25% of patients with advanced diabetic nephropathy. Nodular lesions are an indication of more severe renal damage and poorer prognosis. Classification of diabetic nephropathy depends mainly on glomerular lesions which are responsible for the primary pathology in diabetic nephropathy, although extraglomerular lesions, such as tubulointerstitial lesions are also involved in the progression of the disease. Not all patients with diabetic nephropathy develop proteinuria, with non-proteinuric diabetic nephropathy an increasingly recognised entity.

Other renal disease often coexists with diabetic nephropathy, and nephropathy associated with type 2 diabetes tends to be more complex than that associated with type 1 diabetes.

Hyalinosis of the efferent arteriole is a feature by which diabetic nephropathy could be differentiated from hypertensive nephropathy.[189,190,191]

55.Answer c

Physiological aldosterone synthesis is stimulated by Intravascular volume depletion and/or hyperkalaemia. Intravascular volume depletion causes release of angiotensin II via the renin-angiotensin system which leads to aldosterone release from the zona glomerulosa cells of the adrenal gland.[192,193]

56. Answer c

Resistant hypertension is defined as blood pressure >140/90 in spite of treatment with three antihypertensive agents. Secondary causes should be considered.[192,193]

57. Answer d

Dexamethasone 6mg daily has been shown to reduce mortality in those with COVID-19 requiring ventilatory support and in those requiring supplemental oxygen. It has not been shown to be of value in early mild disease.[194]

58. Answer a

Zidovudine, also known as azidothymidine (AZT) was licenced in the USA in 1987. It is a reverse transcriptase inhibitor. It led to modest improvements in those with HIV. Subsequent improvements in HIV outcomes arose with the use of two-drug and especially three-drug anti-retroviral treatment regimens.[197]

59. Answer e

Cervical spondylosis refers to progressive osseocartilaginous deterioration of the cervical spine usually related to aging. It is more common in men. Radiculopathy or myelopathy leading to neurological symptoms and signs occur in a minority. Population based studies have shown that 80-90% of people will have some element of cervical disc degeneration on MRI scan by the age of 50 years. In a global review in 2015 more than a third of a billion people worldwide had mechanical neck pain of more than 3 months duration at some point. Degenerative changes of the spine may occur as early as the first decade of life.[198]

60. Answer b

Chronic lymphocytic leukaemia is a malignancy of CD5+ lymphocytes characterised by accumulation of small, mature-appearing lymphocytes in the blood, bone marrow and secondary lymphoid tissues.[199,200]

61. Answer a

Respiratory failure occurs due to a failure of ventilation (movement of gas in and out of the lungs) or gas exchange (transferring oxygen from air to blood and transferring carbon dioxide from blood to air).

Type 1 respiratory failure occurs when there is hypoxia with normal or low carbon dioxide in the blood (<6kPa). It represents a failure of gas exchange, with the increased solubility of carbon dioxide in the blood preventing hypercapnia.

Type 2 respiratory failure occurs when there is hypoxia with high carbon dioxide in the blood (>6kPa). It represents a failure of lung ventilation with or without failure of gas exchange.

Pneumonia, heart failure, severe COVID-19 and pulmonary embolus cause respiratory failure usually due their effects on gas exchange rather than causing hypoventilation. Respiratory failure due to opiate toxicity will cause hypoventilation and hypercapnia.[214]

62. Answer d

Lung cancer staging is essential for determining appropriate treatment in both small cell and non-small cell lung cancer. Surgical resection is potentially curative in stages IA, IB, IIA and IIB non-small cell lung cancer. This indicates a primary tumour of maximum size 5cm with localised nodal involvement (T2BN1), or up to 7cm with no nodal involvement (T3N0M0).[201,202,203]

63. Answer c

Pulmonary hypertension is a severe vascular disorder defined as mean pulmonary arterial pressure of 25mmHg or more at rest. Pulmonary arterial hypertension describes a subgroup with pulmonary arterial pressure of 25mmHg or greater as well as normal pulmonary capillary wedge pressure of 15mmHg or less and pulmonary vascular resistance of greater than 3 Wood units, and where other common causes of pulmonary hypertension such as chronic lung disease, chronic pulmonary thromboembolic disease or left heart failure are not present.[204,205]

64. Answer c

Diagnosis of hereditary haemorrhagic telangiectasia (HHT) can be made by genetic testing or by using the Curacao criteria. These criteria are

- recurrent and spontaneous epistaxis
- visceral localisation
- an affected first degree family member
- mucocutaneous telangiectasia

Three or more criteria indicates HHT, the presence of two indicates possible HHT and the presence of none or one indicates unlikely HHT.[204]

65. Answer e

70-80% of mesotheliomas arise from the pleura with the remainder mostly involving the peritoneum. Pericardial mesothelioma is rare. Mesothelioma overall remains a relatively rare cancer (incidence rate 1 per 100,000 in the US and 1-3 per 100,000 in Europe).[206]

66. Answer d

Psoriasis may be triggered by medications in those with or without a history of psoriasis. There are a long list of drugs linked to psoriasis but most are case reports only. Strong evidence for a link with psoriasis exists only for betablockers, lithium and tumour necrosis factor alpha antagonists, which have been assessed in large cohort and case-control studies. The latency period may be up to 12 months in particular for lithium and betablockers.

Psoriasis may not resolve on discontinuation of the medication. Drug-induced psoriasis will not be clinically distinguishable from other forms of psoriasis. There may be histological differences (lack of tortuous papillary dermal capillaries and associated suprapapillary epidermal thinning) but these differences may not be present. The initial treatment is removal of the offending drug, but this is not always possible. Treatment with usual topical or systemic treatments may be effective.[207]

67. Answer a

Wilson's disease occurs due to mutation to the ATP7B gene which encodes a transmembrane copper-transporting ATPase.

Mutations in the other genes listed are involved in hereditary haemochromatosis.[208]

68. Answer c

Drugs are one of the most common causes of hyponatraemia. Thiazide and loop diuretics (thiazides more frequently), SSRIs, SNRIs, phenothiazines, tricyclic antidepressants, NSAIDs, proton pump inhibitors and ACE inhibitors among others. Lithium is associated with nephrogenic diabetes insipidus (occurring in 15% of those on lithium) usually causing hypernatraemia. Conversely, nephrogenic diabetes insipidus may also occur in those taking loop diuretics or nephrotoxic drugs.[209,210]

69. Answer a

Anosmia is loss of sense of smell and may be conductive (physical barriers preventing odorants reaching the olfactory system) or central (problems with the olfactory system detecting odorants). It occurs in 20% of adults and up to 80% of those over the age of 75.

It occurs in around one half of patients with COVID-19 and may be associated with loss of taste. It resolves in 90% of these patients within four weeks.

It requires investigation if persistent for 6 weeks, or for three months in those with a positive COVID-19 test.

Central causes such as meningioma of the olfactory groove are rare but should be considered.[211]

70. Answer c

Bacillus Calmette-Guerin (BCG) vaccination is a live attenuated form of Mycobacterium bovis. It is used to protect against tuberculosis. It also offers protection against non-tuberculous mycobacteria infections such as leprosy and Buruli ulcer. It is used in the treatment of superficial bladder cancer. It forms part of the childhood immunisation regime in many countries, but current WHO guidance recommends routine neonatal vaccination only in countries with moderate to severe prevalence of tuberculosis.

Disseminated BCG infection has been described after vaccination in the immunosuppressed, and after bladder cancer treatment, and may not emerge for many years.[215,216,217]

71. Answer c

Staphylococcus aureus is the cause of native valve endocarditis in 30-40% of cases. Streptococcus viridans is a cause in about 20% if cases. Coagulase negative staphylococcus is a common cause of prosthetic valve endocarditis but uncommon in native valve endocarditis.[218]

72. Answer e

Diagnostic criteria for polymyalgia rheumatica involves a scoring system in those with symptoms and raised inflammatory markers, with points allocated for morning stiffness for more than 45 minutes, hip pain or limited range of motion, absence of rheumatoid factor or anti-citrullinated protein antibody, absence of other joint involvement and radiological signs of subdeltoid bursitis, biceps tenosynovitis, glenohumeral synovitis, hip synovitis or trochanteric bursitis.[219,220,221]

73. Answer e

Postural tachycardia syndrome (POTS) is a syndrome characterised by chronic symptoms of orthostatic intolerance with sustained and excessive sinus tachycardia in the absence of orthostatic hypotension. Symptoms of orthostatic intolerance may include palpitations, chest pain or discomfort, lightheadedness, blurred vision, dyspnoea, headache, nausea and fatigue.

Syncope may occur but is not required for diagnosis. Diagnosis depends on the chronicity of symptoms and the demonstration of an increase in heart rate of 30 bpm or more on standing. Tilt table is not needed for diagnosis and may be less clinically relevant than demonstrating tachycardia on normal standing. POTS may affect quality of life but there is no increase in mortality.[222]

74. Answer e

Joint hypermobility refers to excessive mobility of joints. It may be localised or generalised (generalised joint hypermobility) and is assessed using the Beighton score involving five clinical manoeuvres. It is a clinical finding rather than a disease and is often asymptomatic. Joint hypermobility syndrome refers to generalised joint hypermobility and chronic musculoskeletal pain. There is considerable overlap with heritable connective tissue disorders such as Marfan syndrome, osteogenesis imperfecta and especially Ehlers Danlos syndrome. The Brighton criteria are used to diagnose joint hypermobility syndrome and the Villefranche criteria are used to diagnose Ehlers Danlos syndrome. Neither condition has been linked with a specific genetic cause and as both have considerable clinical overlap they are considered by some to be the same condition.[223]

75. Answer a

Trigeminal neuralgia is sudden, intense and short paroxysms of pain in the territory of one or more divisions of the trigeminal nerve. It is a clinical diagnosis, although MRI scan should be performed to exclude secondary causes. Bilateral pain is rare and alternative diagnoses should be considered if this occurs. 91-99% of those with trigeminal neuralgia report pain triggered by innocuous stimuli on the face or intraoral trigeminal territory. The second (maxillary) and third (mandibular) divisions are most often affected.

Even though paroxysmal pain is the hallmark of trigeminal neuralgia 24-49% of patients describe continuous pain between paroxysmal attacks.[224]

76. Answer a

Post-acute COVID-19 symptoms (or long COVID-19) are symptoms lasting beyond three weeks in those with a diagnosis of COVID-19 The array of symptoms at the time of writing is enormous. The most common are cough, low grade fever and fatigue, but many symptoms are described. The challenge facing physicians lies in identifying mild symptoms likely to resolve from those indicating a serious COVID-19 complication such as pericarditis or pulmonary embolus.[225]

77. Answer e

Colour deficiency is one of the most common visual problems and can be divided into acquired or congenital. Congenital colour deficiency is usually X-linked and most commonly affects red-green colour vision. 'Red-green colour deficiency' is a term which encompasses an array of X-linked recessive traits which causes defects in red and green vision to varying degrees. These traits (known as protanomaly, deuteranomaly, protanopia, deuteranopia) are the most common forms of congenital colour vision deficiency. Humans are trichromatic, which means that they can perceive combinations of three primary colours. There are three types of cone (not rod) photoreceptors involving different wavelengths of light and colour vision depending on how these signals are interpreted by the central nervous system. Congenital colour vision deficiency tends to involve genetic mutations which lead to abnormal functioning of cone photoreceptors. Up to 8% of males and 0.5% of females may be affected, with Europeans affected more commonly than Africans.[226,227]

78. Answer e

Thyroid nodules are common and often detected incidentally on radiology performed for another reason. Autopsy studies report that they are present in 50-60% of adults. They are more common with advancing age and in women. Most are benign, the rate of malignancy is uncertain but likely to be between 1.6% and 12%. Ultrasound is the best modality for measuring size and assessing for signs of malignancy. Microcalcifications, hypoechogenicity, irregular margins and shape taller than wide on transverse view are all ultrasound features suggestive of malignancy in thyroid nodules.[228,229]

79. Answer d

Carbon monoxide (CO) poisoning is a difficult diagnosis due to its non specific presentation. Carbon monoxide displaces oxygen from haemoglobin forming carboxyhaemoglobin. Smokers may have an increased tolerance to CO so symptoms may only appear after substantial exposure. Carboxyhaemoglobin has a brighter hue than oxyhaemoglobin but the 'cherry red' skin described in CO poisoning probably exists only in textbooks. Oxygen saturation is often falsely high due to the similar properties of oxyhaemoglobin and carboxyhaemoglobin.

Venous blood levels of carboxyhaemoglobin of 15-20% will cause toxicity and treatment is by displacing carbon monoxide with 100% oxygen.[230]

80. Answer b

Primary biliary cirrhosis is an autoimmune disorder of the liver characterised by chronic biochemical cholestasis, positive anti-mitochondrial antibodies and liver histology showing nonsuppurative destructive cholangitis and interlobular bile duct destruction. Women are affected ten-fold more frequently than men, Recurrent urinary tract infections, cigarette smoking and a positive family history are also risk factors. Alcohol intake has been negatively associated with risk.[231]

81. Answer c

QT interval was not seen as a significant source of pathology when ECG waveforms were described first in the late 19th century. The discovery in the 1950s and 1960s of families of children with recurring syncope, sudden childhood death and long QT intervals on ECG led to the recognition of congenital long QT syndrome.

Congenital long QT syndromes are characterised by syncopal episodes and sudden death. All associated genes encode cardiac ion channel subunits or proteins involved in modulating ionic currents.

Some of the children originally described also had congenital deafness, subsequently identified as Jervell-Lange-Nielson syndrome. Romano Ward syndrome is congenital long QT syndrome without congenital deafness.[232,233]

82. Answer c

Pregabalin is an anticonvulsant medication that has been repurposed as an analgesic and anxiety medication. It is licensed for neuropathic pain and generalised anxiety disorder, and as an add-on therapy in partial epilepsy. It also has a licence for the treatment of fibromyalgia in the USA. Its use increased largely due to off-licence use, in spite of a lack of evidence for benefit in nociceptive, post-operative pain, sciatica and migraine. Its benefits in neuropathic pain are modest, with most studies showing a number needed to treat of 6 to 8 to achieve a measured 50% improvement in pain.[234,235,236,237,238]

83. Answer b

Many medical journal opinion pieces have expressed concerns about the use of generic medications despite the lack of evidence of any superiority of originator medications.

Applications for authorisation of generic medicines do not need to show any new pre-clinical or clinical data, but instead focus on ensuring that the generic medicine has pharmacokinetics comparable to the originator product. Such applications generally aim to show bioequivalence to the reference drug. The mandated bioequivalence parameters require adhering to an AUC (area under the curve, which reflects the extent of absorption and exposure to the drug) and C_{max} (maximum plasma concentration) of 80 -125% at a 90% confidence interval, as compared to the reference drug. Without the need for lengthy clinical studies prior to market authorisation generic drug manufacturers can sell their medicines at a discounted price.

There are some concerns around the use of bioequivalence studies. They are performed on relatively small numbers of healthy volunteers. Significant individual pharmacokinetic variations due to medical conditions may be missed, and the focus on averages may not properly evaluate patients with outlier-level drug pharmacokinetics. They may not be relevant to narrow therapeutic index drugs. Due to the 80 to 125% reference-generic bioequivalence standard, there may be significant generic-generic variability resulting so-called generic 'drift', where subsequent generic products differ significantly from the originator.

In spite of these concerns, there are few studies which prove adverse effects of generic medications, and when studied any variation compares favourably to batch-batch variations of branded medications. A review if clinical equivalence studies comparing generic and brand-name drugs in cardiovascular medicines published in JAMA in 2008 found no significant difference between generics and originators.

A position statement published in 2016 by the Amer can Epilepsy Society in 2016 acknowledged that some currently used anticonvulsants such as valproic acid and carbamazepine are themselves generic derivatives from originators developed in the 1970s. The statement supports the interchangeability of originator and generic anticonvulsants which have passed the FDA bioequivalence regulations, with certain qualifiers such as avoiding substituting short-release with extended-release products and ensuring patients are aware of any changes in colour or other appearances of their medications. This was largely based on two FDA-funded studies looking at lamotrigine which showed excellent bioequivalence.[240,241,242,243]

84. Answer a

Clostridium difficile, a gram positive, anaerobic, spore-forming, toxin producing bacillus, was officially renamed Clostridioides difficile in 2016, to reflect differences between this species and other members of the clostridium genus. It has been known as a gut commensal for many years, and its association with diarrhoeal infection has increased since the introduction of antibiotics. Nearly every antibiotic has been associated with the development of Clostridioides difficile infection (CDI) including those used in treatment of CDI, vancomycin and metronidazole. The most common antibiotics associated with CDI are broad spectrum penicillins and cephalosporins, clindamycin and flouroquinolones.[244]

85. Answer d

Cholinesterase inhibitors used for the treatment of cementia are associated with increase risk of bradycardia and atrioventricular or sino-atrial block. An ECG should be performed to exclude heart block prior to initiating these medications.[247]

86. Answer c

The HAS-BLED score estimates risk of bleeding on anticoagulation treatment. It gives a point for uncontrolled hypertension, renal disease, liver disease, stroke history, prior major bleeding or predisposition to bleeding, labile INR, age>65 years, use of anti-platelet medication or NSAID and alcohol use.

Dementia is not a risk factor for bleeding on anticoagulation.[248]

87. Answer d

Herpes zoster ophthalmicus occurs when varicella zoster recurrence affects the ophthalmic branch of the trigeminal nerve. Several ophthalmic complications may occur, including keratitis, corneal ulceration, uveitis, scleritis, episcleritis, glaucoma, retinal necrosis and optic neuritis. Keratitis is the most common complication. Acute retinal necrosis is associated with probable permanent visual loss.

Hutchinson sign refers to rash affecting the nose and is highly predictive of ocular involvement.[249]

88. Answer c

Frontotemporal dementia refers to a dementia arising from progressive degeneration of the fontal and anterior temporal lobes and is the most common type of dementia occurring in those under the age of 65 years.[247]

89. Answer b

There are two main types of autoimmune blistering disease: pemphigus and pemphigoid. Pemphigus occurs due to blistering in the epidermis and pemphigoid due to subepidermal blistering.

Pemphigus occurs due to autoantibodies targeting desmoglein 1 and desmoglein 3 (Dsg 1 and Dsg 3) which play a role in desmosomes essential for cell to cell adhesion.

Pemphigoid occurs due to autoantibodies that target components of hemidesmosomes in the basement membrane zone.[250,251,252]

90. Answer d

All of the listed medications have been associated with drug induced autoimmune hepatitis but nitrofurantoin and minocycline are the most common, accounting for 90% of cases worldwide.[257]

91. Answer c

Familial hypercholesterolaemia is a common inherited condition resulting in prolonged exposure to high LDL levels and premature cardiovascular disease in men and women.[258]

92. Answer d

Dix Hallpike manoeuvre is a sensitive and specific test for the diagnosis of benign paroxysmal positional vertigo (BPPV). It is performed with the patient seated with head turned to 45 degrees, then asked to lie back flat. Hanging the head over the back if the bed on lying flat is not necessary. The test is positive with onset of appropriate nystagmus, with is a torsional nystagmus with a latency of onset and limited duration to a few seconds only. The nystagmus will occur in the opposite direction on sitting up straight. Fatiguability of the nystagmus occurs on repeated testing. Intensity of nystagmus correlates with severity of vertigo.[263]

93. Answer e

Scleroderma is a connective tissue disease characterised by micro vascular damage and excessive deposition of collagen in the skin and internal organs. It is divided into a localised form (morphoea) which affects the skin only, and a generalised form known as systemic sclerosis. Systemic sclerosis is further subdivided into limited cutaneous systemic scleroderma (lcSSc or CREST syndrome) and a diffuse cutaneous systemic scleroderma (dcSSc). These have separate clinical features and are associated with different serological positivity. CREST syndrome is associated with positive anticentromere antibodies and dcSSc is associatec with positive antipoisomerase and anti-RNAP III antibodies.[266]

94. Answer b

Guillain Barre syndrome is a progressive motor weakness, usually symmetrical and beginning in the legs, and reaching its maximum weakness within four weeks of onset. It is assumed to be due to an immunological response to triggers such as surgery or infection. There are reduced tendon reflexes or areflexia. Two thirds will have autonomic effects such as cardiac arrhythmia and blood pressure instability. Cerebrospinal fluid shows raised protein levels with normal white cell levels.[267,268]

95. Answer a

Polycystic kidneys are a relatively common cause of end-stage renal disease. They are monogenic cilia-related disorders. Autosomal dominant polycystic kidney disease (ADPKD) is much more common and has a less severe course than autosomal recessive polycystic kidney disease (ARPKD). ARPKD tends to present perinatally or in young children with renal failure. ADPKD usually presents in adults and progresses to end stage renal disease in 75% by the age of 70.[270]

96. Answer e

C-peptide is a by-product of insulin release, so levels reflect the amount of circulating insulin a patient has. It can be useful in distinguishing between type 1 and type 2 diabetes where diagnostic uncertainty exists. However about 30% of patients with type 1 diabetes have detectable C-peptide measurements and has been superseded by testing for autoantibodies to pancreatic β cells or insulin.[273]

97. Answer d

Interferon-γ-release assays (IGRAs) such as the Quantiferon TB-Gold assay are used primarily to detect latent tuberculosis (TB). They offer advantage over tuberculin skin testing (TST) in that they do not cross-react in those who have had previous BCG vaccination. They are also less likely to cross-react with non-tuberculous mycobacteria (NTM) although there may be some cross-reaction with some NTM. They cannot distinguish between active and latent tuberculosis and are poorly predictive of who will progress from latent to active tuberculosis. IGRAs detect interferon-γ secretion by T lymphocytes which are stimulated by TB-specific antigens.[281,282,283]

98. Answer d

Hepatorenal syndrome is renal impairment in those with liver cirrhosis, characterised by a reduction in renal blood flow and glomerular filtration rate. Renal damage can be reversible through liver transplantation or vasoconstrictor drugs. Serum creatinine levels may underestimate renal function deterioration in those with liver cirrhosis due to impaired hepatic production of creatine, reduced muscle mass and other factors. However serum creatinine remains an important marker of renal deterioration in hepatorenal syndrome in the absence of an alternative. Standard definition of acute kidney injury include deterioration in urinary output, but this is less useful in liver cirrhosis where urinary output is already lowered due to sodium and water retention.

Hepatorenal syndrome is subdivided into hepatorena syndrome with acute kidney injury (HRS-AKI) and hepatorenal syndrome with non-acute kidney injury (HRS-NAKI). Diagnosis of HRS-AKI requires deterioration of serum creatinine to a given level within 48 hours and the absence of structural kidney injury reflected in the absence of proteinuria, haematuria and normal renal ultrasound. Hypovolaemia may occur in liver cirrhosis due to a number of factors, leading to acute tubular necrosis, and differentiating this from HRS-AKI can be challenging.

Risk factors for development of AKI-HRS in those with cirrhosis include severity of ascites, liver size, high plasma renin activity and hyponatraemia.[287]

99. Answer d

Gout is the most common inflammatory arthropathy and occurs due to hyperuricaemia and monosodium crystal deposition. A minority of people with hyperuricaemia will develop gout (for example 7% within one year for those with serum uric acid levels >595μmol/L). It is much more common in men, and very uncommon in pre-menopausal women due to protective effects of oestrogen and progesterone. The gender difference decreases over the age of 60. Starting at lower doses of uric acid lowering treatment reduces risk of acute gout flares. As it usually presents as a monoarthritis, the main differential diagnosis is septic arthritis.

Chronic tophaceous gout usually develops after many years of uncontrolled gout. It may develop more quickly in some, including solid organ transplant recipients on low dose prednisolone and calcineurin inhibitors.[288]

100. Answer b

Idiosyncratic drug-induced liver injury occurs when there are alterations in liver biochemical tests resulting from appropriate use of a drug within recommended dosages. It can vary from mild asymptomatic and self-limiting rise in liver biochemical tests to life-threatening acute liver failure. Several drugs are implicated. Anti-microbials are the most common cause worldwide although the specific drugs may vary between different countries, with amoxicillin and flucloxacillin common causes in Europe and anti-tuberculous drugs the most common in India.[294]

1. Trans catheter aortic valve implantation (TAVI):
    a.   Is primarily indicated in younger patients with aortic stenosis
    b.   Is primarily indicated in older patients with aortic stenosis
    c.   Is primarily indicated in patients with aortic stenosis due to bicuspid aortic valve
    d.   Is primarily indicated in those with low operative risk
    e.   Is primarily indicated in those with high operative risk

2. The most common site for arterial thrombosis in anti-phospholipid syndrome (APS) is:
    a.   The heart
    b.   The lower limb
    c.   The brain
    d.   The eye
    e.   The upper limb

3. Spontaneous bacterial peritonitis (SBP):
    a.   Usually has a surgical cause
    b.   Is nearly always symptomatic
    c.   All patients admitted to hospital with decompensated liver failure and ascites should have an ascitic tap to exclude SBP
    d.   An ascitic fluid polymorphonuclear count of $>5/mm^3$ is considered diagnostic of SBP
    e.   Ascitic culture should be awaited prior to starting antibiotics in suspected SBP

4. The proportion of duodenal ulcers associated with Helicobacter pylori is:
    a.   10%
    b.   30%
    c.   50%
    d.   70%
    e.   90%

5. ACE inhibitor-induced angioedema:
- a. Being African-American is a risk factor
- b. Is more common in men
- c. Is more common in non-smokers
- d. Will not occur after the medication has been discontinued
- e. The medication can usually be continued once the angioedema is treated

6. Lyme disease:
- a. Erythema migrans is a spreading rash seen in Lyme disease but it is not diagnostic
- b. The erythema migrans rash usually appears and disappears within 48 hours of a tick bite
- c. Erythema migrans is not usually itchy, hot or painful
- d. Lyme disease does not have a seasonal occurrence
- e. Negative Lyme serology excludes a diagnosis of Lyme disease

7. The most common cause of morbidity and mortality in Marfan syndrome is:
- a. Mitral valve regurgitation
- b. Endocarditis
- c. Spontaneous pneumothorax
- d. Aortic root disease
- e. Abdominal aortic aneurysm

8. Peak expiratory flow rate is:
- a. The maximum rate of airflow achieved during expiration starting at full inspiration with an open glottis
- b. The maximum amount of air that can be expelled from the lungs during a forced expiration from a position of full inspiration
- c. The maximum amount of air that can be expelled from the lungs in the first second of a forced expiration from a position of full inspiration
- d. The maximum amount of air which can be exhaled or inspired during a forced or slow manoeuvre
- e. The average expired flow over the middle half of a forced expiratory manoeuvre manoeuvre

9. Which of the following is associated with low risk of progression in monoclonal gammopathy of undetermined significance (MGUS):
    a.   Low level of M protein <1.5g/dl
    b.   IgM type MGUS
    c.   Kappa-lambda light chain ratio <0.26
    d.   Kappa-lambda light chain ratio >1.65
    e.   5% progression to myeloma per year

10. Dengue fever:
    a.   Is spread by the Anopheles mosquito
    b.   May progress to haemorrhagic fever
    c.   Infection will confer lifelong immunity to Dengue
    d.   Most deaths occur in the elderly
    e.   Can be treated with anti-viral medication

11. Raynaud's phenomenon:
    a.   Affects only the fingers
    b.   The colour change sequence is blue-white-red
    c.   Primary Raynaud's is more likely to lead to complications than secondary Raynaud's
    d.   Nailfold capillaroscopy can differentiate between primary and secondary Raynaud's
    e.   There is no evidence for the use of calcium channel blockers in treatment

12. Which of the following is the odd one out, with regard to its mosquito vector:
    a.   Zika virus
    b.   Chikungunya virus
    c.   Malaria
    d.   Yellow fever
    e.   Dengue

13. Most cases of statin intolerance resulting in discontinuation are due to:
   a.   Headache
   b.   Laboratory abnormalities
   c.   Erectile dysfunction
   d.   Dyspepsia
   e.   Statin associated muscle symptoms

14. Axial spondyloarthropathies:
   a.   Affect men more than women
   b.   Do not occur in individuals who are HLA B 27 negative
   c.   Can be ruled out in an individual with a normal MRI scan of lumbosacral spine
   d.   Cause low back pain that worsens with movement
   e.   May cause blindness

15. The most common monogenic disorder is:
   a.   Cystic fibrosis
   b.   Sickle cell disease
   c.   Marfan syndrome
   d.   Haemochromatosis
   e.   Haemophilia

16. Tuberculosis (TB):
   a.   Genito-urinary TB may be communicable
   b.   Multi-drug resistant TB (MDR-TB) refers to TB resistant to rifampicin
   c.   Latent TB present for over two years is at higher risk of re-activation than disease present for less then two years
   d.   Interferon gamma release assays have sensitivity and specificity of 85-90% for mycobacterium tuberculosis detection
   e.   Lifetime risk of reactivation of latent TB is 50%

17. Neurosarcoidosis:
a. Usually presents without other systems being affected by sarcoid
b. May cause blindness
c. Affects only the cranial nerves
d. Facial palsy is usually permanent
e. Usually resolves spontaneously without treatment

18. The most common cause of right ventricular failure is:
a. Left ventricular failure
b. Pulmonary embolus
c. Chronic lung disease
d. Tricuspid regurgitation
e. Myocarditis

19. McDonald criteria (2017) for diagnosing multiple sclerosis:
a. Are used primarily to differentiate multiple sclerosis from other diagnoses
b. Are used primarily to diagnose multiple sclerosis in those with clinically isolated syndrome
c. Require cerebrospinal fluid analysis is most cases to diagnose multiple sclerosis
d. Are not used in progressive multiple sclerosis
e. More than one MRI scan is always needed to demonstrate dissemination in time

20. Penicillin allergy:
a. Is always lifelong
b. Precludes the use of cephalosporins
c. Is associated with a reduced risk of methicillin resistant staphylococcus aureus (MRSA) colonisation
d. Up to 90% of those labelled with penicillin allergy may be able to safely take penicillin
e. Oral re-challenge of penicillin can be tried at home for those suspected to have been mis-labelled with penicillin allergy

21. Drug reaction with eosinophilia and systemic symptoms (DRESS syndrome):
    a. Eosinophilia is universal
    b. The heart is the most common non-dermatological organ involved
    c. Mortality is 50%
    d. Facial oedema is a useful clinical characteristic for diagnosis
    e. The rash is typically urticarial

22. Which of the following is not a known adverse effect of methotrexate:
    a. Osteoporosis
    b. Liver fibrosis
    c. Skin nodulosis
    d. Alopecia
    e. Stomatitis

23. Atrial fibrillation and stroke risk:
    a. Stroke risk is higher in males than females
    b. Stroke risk is higher in those with heart failure with reduced ejection fraction than with preserved ejection fraction
    c. Stroke risk is higher in non-valvular atrial fibrillation than valvular atrial fibrillation
    d. Stroke risk is higher in non-diabetics than diabetics
    e. Stroke risk is higher in uncontrolled hypertension than controlled hypertension

24. Parkinson's disease:
    a. Does not present under the age of 50
    b. Occurs sporadically and cannot be inherited
    c. First degree relatives of an individual with Parkinson's disease are not at increased risk of developing the disease
    d. MRI brain is useful in the diagnosis of Parkinson's disease
    e. The lifetime cumulative risk for developing Parkinson's disease in the general population is 4%

25. Complications of coeliac disease:
    a. Are more likely the younger the age of diagnosis of coeliac disease
    b. Are less common in seronegative coeliac disease
    c. Hyposplenism occurs in all individuals with coeliac disease
    d. Intestinal lymphoma usually develops in those with refractory coeliac disease
    e. Small bowel adenocarcinoma is the most common gastrointestinal malignancy in coeliac disease

26. Which of the following is not a typical clinical feature of Cushing syndrome:
    a. Hypoglycaemia
    b. Proximal muscle wasting
    c. Easy bruising
    d. Acne
    e. Susceptibility to infection

27. The most commonly isolated respiratory pathogen in cystic fibrosis is:
    a. Staphylococcus aureus
    b. Haemophilus influenza
    c. Pseudomonas aeruginosa
    d. Streptococcus pneumonia
    e. Moraxella catarrhalis

28. The Vaughan Williams class of flecainide is:
    a. IA
    b. IC
    c. II
    d. III
    e. IV

29. Lipids:
   a.   The relationship between LDL reduction and reduced cardiovascular risk is non-linear
   b.   For every reduction of 39 mg/dl (1.0 mmol/L) in LDL cholesterol level, statins confer relative reductions in all-cause mortality of 30%
   c.   PCSK9 inhibitors have been shown to reduce cardiovascular events by 15%
   d.   Ezetimibe does not increase hepatic LDL receptor expression
   e.   Long-chain n–3 polyunsaturated fatty acids have been shown to reduce cardiovascular events and mortality

30. The most common sites for presentation of painless enlargement of adenopathy in Hodgkin's lymphoma are:
   a.   Mediastinum and spleen
   b.   Mediastinum and neck
   c.   Abdominal and neck
   d.   Abdominal and inguinofemoral area
   e.   Neck and inguinofemoral area

31. Which of the following is not a risk factor for recurrence in an individual with venous thromboembolic disease (deep vein thrombosis or pulmonary embolism):
   a.   Distal DVT
   b.   Post thrombotic limb syndrome
   c.   Advanced age
   d.   Unprovoked DVT
   e.   Unprovoked PE

32. Filoviruses:
   a.   Are spherical
   b.   Are DNA viruses
   c.   Are zoonotic pathogens
   d.   Do not cause fatal disease
   e.   Spread occurs by mucous membrane spread only and will not occur percutaneously

33. Which of the following medications are most useful for reducing mortality in heart failure with preserved ejection fraction (HFpEF):
    a. Loop diuretics
    b. ACE inhibitors
    c. Mineralocorticoid receptor antagonists
    d. Betablockers
    e. No medications are shown to reduce mortality in HFpEF

34. Fournier's gangrene:
    a. Occurs only in men
    b. Is rarely fatal
    c. Is characterised by a cellulitis of the perineal, perianal and genital areas
    d. Is usually idiopathic
    e. Early surgical intervention can improve outcome

35. Intestinal inflammation in ulcerative colitis usually begins in the:
    a. Terminal ileum
    b. Anal canal
    c. Sigmoid colon
    d. Proximal colon
    e. Rectum

36. Infective endocarditis:
    a. The average age of those affected has decreased in the past 100 years
    b. 50% of cases will develop a positive rheumatoid factor
    c. May occur in native valves without bacteraemia
    d. Is most commonly caused by gram-negative bacteria
    e. Antibiotic prophylaxis to prevent infective endocarditis after dental extraction has been demonstrated to be effective in randomised controlled trials

37. Which of the following is least likely to occur in a transient ischaemic attack:
    a.   Unilateral facial and arm weakness
    b.   Unilateral arm and leg weakness
    c.   Transient loss of consciousness
    d.   Homonymous hemianopia
    e.   Dysarthria

38. The specificity of a test refers to:
    a.   The proportion of people with a condition who have a positive test result
    b.   The proportion of people without a condition who have a negative test result
    c.   The proportion of people with a condition who have a negative test result
    d.   The proportion of people without a condition who have a positive test result
    e.   The proportion of people with a condition with a given test result (either positive or negative) divided by the proportion of people without the condition with that result

39. Hypersensitivity pneumonitis:
    a.   Is a type 1 hypersensitivity reaction
    b.   Is a granulomatous disease
    c.   Corticosteroids will reduce progression of the disease
    d.   Chemical worker's lung is the most common form
    e.   Will not affect children

40. The most common side effect of acitretin is:
    a.   Conjunctivitis
    b.   Cheilitis
    c.   Effluvium
    d.   Hepatitis
    e.   Teratogenicity

41. Teriparatide:

a. Is a truncated calcitonin analogue
b. Is a truncated parathyroid hormone analogue
c. Reduces vertebral fracture risk out not hip fracture risk
d. Is associated with increased risk of osteosarcoma in humans
e. Is licenced for use in osteoporosis for up to 5 years

42. Hepatitis C virus infection:

a. 90% of those with chronic hepatitis C virus infection will develop liver cirrhosis
b. Antibody testing can distinguish between acute and chronic hepatitis C infection
c. Antibody testing can distinguish those who have spontaneously cleared the virus from those with chronic infection
d. Those who have had successful antivirus treatment and have cleared the virus will have a positive antibody test
e. Sexual transmission is the most common form of transmission of hepatitis C virus

43. Rheumatoid factor antibodies are:

a. IgM antibodies
b. IgA antibodies
c. IgG antibodies
d. IgE antibodies
e. Light chains

44. Common variable immunodeficiency:

a. There is increased risk of autoimmune disorders
b. B cell levels are usually reduced
c. Identified monogenic mutations account for 90% of cases
d. There is increased incidence of Helicobacter pylori infection
e. Immunoglobulin treatment improves gastrointestinal treatments

45. The most common chromosomal condition associated with intellectual disability is:
    a.   Williams syndrome
    b.   Down syndrome
    c.   Turner syndrome
    d.   Prader Willi syndrome
    e.   Noonan syndrome

46. Thrombophilia:
    a.   Acquired thrombophilias are more likely to cause arterial thrombosis than inherited thrombophilias
    b.   All patients diagnosed with venous thromboembolic disease should have thrombophilia testing
    c.   Testing for Factor V Leiden will be unreliable during an acute venous thromboembolic event
    d.   Inherited thrombophilia is more common in those of African descent
    e.   Bechet's disease is the most common form of acquired thrombophilia

47. Acute intermittent porphyria:
    a.   Exogenous oestrogens may precipitate attacks
    b.   Rash is the most common manifestation of acute attacks
    c.   Most of those with the genetic mutation will develop acute attacks
    d.   Attacks are not life-threatening
    e.   Blue urine is a feature of attacks

48. Hyperthyroidism:
    a.   Excess exogenous thyroid hormone intake may lead to hyperthyroidism
    b.   Hyperthyroidism is more likely to occur in iodine sufficient areas
    c.   The incidence of hyperthyroidism decreases with age
    d.   Hyperthyroidism is more common in men
    e.   Toxic nodular goitre and solitary toxic adenoma are more likely to be a cause of hyperthyroidism in iodine deficient areas than in iodine sufficient areas

49. Primary aldosteronism:

    a.   Does not increase mortality risk

    b.   Angiotensin II to renin ratio can be used in screening for primary aldosteronism

    c.   All those with adrenal incidentalomas should be screened for primary aldosteronism

    d.   A glucose tolerance test should be used as a confirmatory test

    e.   Radiology is not required in the management work up

50. Hereditary haemorrhagic telangiectasia:

    a.   Is an autosomal recessive condition

    b.   Gastrointestinal bleeding is the most common symptom

    c.   Is commonly associated with pulmonary hypertension

    d.   Telangiectasias arise due to precapillary vessel dilatation

    e.   Affected family members may have different levels of disease severity

51. Wilson's disease:

    a.   Is rarely fatal even without treatment

    b.   Is autosomal dominant

    c.   Most commonly affects the neurclogical system

    d.   Serum ceruloplasmin levels are always low

    e.   May present with acute liver failure in young females

52. Osmotic demyelination syndrome occurs due to overly rapid correction of serum:

    a.   Calcium

    b.   Sodium

    c.   Potassium

    d.   Glucose

    e.   Protein

53. Chest x ray in COVID-19:

a. Chest x ray is indicated in all patients with COVID-19
b. A normal chest x-ray excludes COVID-19 pneumonia
c. Radiological changes in COVID-19 typically affect the peripheral and lower zones on chest x ray in COVID-19 pneumonia
d. Ground glass opacifications are specific for COVID-19 pneumonia
e. Horizontal linear opacities are specific for COVID-19 pneumonia

54. Polymyalgia rheumatica:

a. Is the most common inflammatory disease in the elderly
b. Should be treated with prednisolone 12-25mg per day initially
c. Prednisolone doses should be stopped within a period of four weeks after starting initial treatment
d. 80% of patients will also have giant cell arteritis
e. Absence of ultrasound evidence of bursitis, synovitis and tenosynovitis suggests a positive diagnosis

55. Which of the following is not a clinical manoeuvre on the Beighton score for evaluation of joint hypermobility:

a. Passive dorsiflexion of the 5th finger more than 90 degrees
b. Passive flexion of the thumb to the forearm
c. Passive flexion of the wrist to the forearm
d. Hyperextension of the elbow to more than 10 degrees
e. Forward flexion of the trunk with knees fully extended and palms resting on the floor

56. Trigeminal neuralgia:

a. Incidence decreases with advancing age
b. Location of paroxysmal pain will be in the same location as the innocuous trigger
c. Pain will not affect the skin overlying the angle of the mandible
d. Pain may occur in areas not supplied by the trigeminal nerve
e. Is most commonly caused by intracranial vascular compression of the trigeminal nerve root

57. Which of the following are <u>not</u> features suggestive of malignancy on ultrasound of a thyroid nodule:
    a. Spongiform appearance of nodule
    b. Microcalcifications
    c. Hypoechogenicity
    d. Irregular margins
    e. Shape taller than wide on transverse view

58. QT interval is measured:
    a. From the end of the QRS complex to the beginning of the T wave
    b. From the end of the QRS complex to the end of the T wave
    c. From the peak of the QRS complex to the beginning of the T wave
    d. From the beginning of the QRS complex to the beginning of the T wave
    e. From the beginning of the QRS complex to the end of the T wave

59. Clostridioides difficile:
    a. Is a sphere-shaped organism
    b. Does not form spores
    c. Is gram negative
    d. Is anaerobic
    e. Does not produce a toxin

60. Upper extremity deep vein thrombosis:
    a. Accounts for 50% of all deep vein thrombosis
    b. Will not lead to a pulmonary embolus
    c. Will not lead to post-thrombotic syndrome of the arm
    d. Secondary UEDVT most commonly occurs due to inherited thrombophilia
    e. Is associated with strenuous muscular effort of the upper limbs

61. Which of the following is most likely to be found on brain imaging in typical Alzheimer's disease:
    a. Occipital lobe atrophy
    b. Fronto-parietal lobe atrophy
    c. Medial temporal and parietal lobe atrophy
    d. Cerebellar atrophy
    e. Negative amyloid PET scan

62. 'Non-valvular' atrial fibrillation refers to atrial fibrillation in somebody who:
    a. Does not have moderate to severe mitral regurgitation or mechanical heart valves
    b. Does not have moderate to severe aortic regurgitation or mechanical heart valves
    c. Does not have moderate to severe mitral stenosis or mechanical heart valves
    d. Does not have moderate to severe aortic stenosis or mechanical heart valves
    e. Does not have any significant valvular heart disease or mechanical heart valves

63. The immune marker with the highest diagnostic sensitivity in adult onset type 2 diabetes mellitus is:
    a. Zinc transporter 8 autoantibodies (ZnT8Ab)
    b. Islet cell cytoplasmic autoantibodies (ICA)
    c. Anti-glutamic acid decarboxylase autoantibodies (anti-GAD)
    d. Insulin autoantibodies (IAA)
    e. Insulinoma-associated 2 autoantibodies (IA2)

64. Sjogren's syndrome:
    a. Diagnosis is excluded if anti-Ro and anti-La antibodies are negative
    b. Rheumatoid factor is negative
    c. Salivary gland biopsy is not helpful
    d. Genital dryness is not a feature
    e. There is increased incidence of developing non-Hodgkin B cell lymphoma

65. Herpes zoster (shingles):
   a. Occurs in the distribution of only one dermatome
   b. Will not affect an indivicual more tnan once
   c. Rash will always occur
   d. May affect internal organs
   e. Never affects the central nervous system

66. Todd paralysis:
   a. Is often permanent
   b. Tends to occur after generalised seizures as well as focal seizures
   c. Is of no value in determining the hemisphere of seizure onset
   d. Duration of paralysis reflects duration of seizure
   e. Is characterised by a generalised paralysis of all limbs

67. Dementia with Lewy bodies:
   a. Dementia may occur year after the development of parkinsonism
   b. Parkinsonism may be absent
   c. Visual hallucinations are common
   d. Attention and alertness are preserved
   e. Cholinesterase inhibitors are contraindicated

68. Autoantibodies targeting desmoglein 1 and desmoglein 3 (Dsg 1 and Dsg 3) lead to blistering in:
   a. Pemphigus
   b. Pemphigoid
   c. Allergic contact dermatitis
   d. Dermatitis herpetiformis
   e. Herpes zoster

69. Inhaled corticosteroids in COPD:
    a.   Are contraindicated
    b.   May decrease mortality
    c.   May decrease exacerbations
    d.   May decrease pneumonia risk
    e.   Should not be given in a combination inhaler

70. Scleroderma:
    a.   Causes excess deposition of elastin in the skin and internal organs
    b.   Localised scleroderma is confined to the skin only
    c.   Diffuse cutaneous systemic scleroderma is associated with positive anti centromere antibodies
    d.   Asbestos exposure is associated with increased risk of scleroderma
    e.   Skin biopsy is required for diagnosis

71. Which of the following is not a criterion on the Wells score for assessment of DVT:
    a.   Cancer treatment or palliation in the past 6 months
    b.   Entire leg swollen
    c.   Previous DVT
    d.   Paralysis, paresis or recent plaster immobilisation of lower limb
    e.   Focal calf erythema

72. Autoimmune hepatitis:
    a.   Cirrhosis is present in one third of patients at diagnosis
    b.   Higher levels of transaminases reflect more severe disease histologically
    c.   Is rarely fatal even if untreated
    d.   Does not occur in men
    e.   The diagnosis is excluded if IgG levels are normal

73. Family hypercholesterolaemia is primarily a disorder of:
a. Increased total cholesterol synthesis
b. Increased total LDL synthesis
c. Decreased HDL synthesis
d. Increased HDL uptake by receptors
e. Reduced LDL uptake by LDL receptors

74. Jacksonian march seizure refers to:
a. Collapse with loss of consciousness and repeated short contractions of various muscle groups
b. Repeated short contractions of various muscle groups lasting less than 1 to 2 seconds
c. Sustained contractions of various muscle groups lasting more than 5 to 10 seconds resulting in posturing of the limbs and whole body
d. Sustained, forceful, involuntary turning of the head and eyes to one side due to tonic contraction of the head and eye muscles
e. Repetitive contractions in one hand progressing up one arm and to the ipsilateral foot and leg

75. The investigation most useful in diagnosis of pulmonary fibrosis is:
a. Pulmonary function testing
b. Serological testing
c. High resolution CT scan
d. Bronchoscopy
e. Chest x ray

76. Darier disease:
a. Hyperkeratotic plaques develop in the seborrheic and intertriginous areas
b. Secondary infection of lesions is rare
c. Friction will not affect the disease
d. Sun exposure will not affect the disease
e. Oral mucosa is not involved

77. Complex regional pain syndrome (CRPS):

a.   Pain tends to occur in a dermatomal distribution
b.   Swelling and colour change are not a feature
c.   Is not associated with an identifiable nerve injury
d.   Fracture of the upper limb is the injury most vulnerable to developing CRPS
e.   Proximal limb fractures are more vulnerable to CRPS than distal limb fractures

78. The most common cause of vertigo is:

a.   Benign paroxysmal positional vertigo
b.   Vertiginous migraine
c.   Multiple sclerosis
d.   Meniere's disease
e.   Viral labyrinthitis

79. Mixed connective tissue disease:

a.   Anti CCP antibodies are required for diagnosis
b.   Features of SLE, systemic sclerosis, polymyositis and rheumatoid arthritis tend to present simultaneously
c.   Raynaud's phenomenon does not occur
d.   Arthritis is the most common clinical feature
e.   Pulmonary hypertension is the most common disease related cause of death

80. GuillainBarre syndrome (GBS):

a.   Occurs in 1 in 100 Campylobacter jejuni infections
b.   Sensory symptoms do not occur
c.   Pain is an early symptom
d.   The sural nerve should always undergo nerve conduction testing in GBS
e.   Cranial nerves are not affected

81. Autosomal dominant polycystic kidney disease (ADPKD):
a. Mutations in PKD2 are responsible for 80% of cases
b. Has a more severe course in women
c. Progression to end stage renal disease is rare
d. 50% of those affected have no family history of ADPKD
e. Hypertension may develop in children with ADPKD

82. Von Willebrand's disease:
a. Genotyping is necessary for diagnosis
b. Von Willebrand factor levels may be normal
c. Von Willebrand factor levels below 50IU per decilitre are sufficient for diagnosis
d. Is most commonly autosomal recessive
e. Factor VIII activity is always reduced

83. Mosaicism:
a. Is the presence of more than one genotype in one individual
b. Is the presence of different manifestations of a particular genotype in one individual
c. Is the presence of different manifestations of a particular genotype in one family
d. Is the presence of different manifestations of a genotype in one organ or system
e. Is the presence of different genetic mutations in first degree relatives

84. Diabetes mellitus:
a. 40% of new cases of type 1 diabetes occur in patients over the age of 30 years of age
b. 2 hour post-glucose challenge plasma glucose of greater than 7.0mmol/L (126mg/dL) is sufficient for diagnosis
c. Random plasma glucose cannot be used for diagnosis
d. HbA1c cannot be used for diagnosis
e. All patients require a glucose tolerance test for diagnosis

85. Those with end-stage renal disease are at risk of a life-threatening syndrome of microvessel calcification and occlusion of the skin and subcutaneous tissue that results in painful necrotic skin lesions, known as:
    a. Dactylitis
    b. Calciphylaxis
    c. Necrotising fasciitis
    d. Erythema gangrenosum
    e. Calcinosis

86. Which of the following is not sufficient for a diagnosis of chronic kidney disease:
    a. History of renal transplantation
    b. Rise in creatinine 1.5 times above baseline
    c. Glomerular filtration rate <60 ml/min/1.73m^2
    d. Protein-to-creatinine ratio of >200mg/g for three months
    e. Albumin-to-creatinine ratio of >30g/g for three months

87. Caplan's syndrome is the association of a pneumoconiosis with:
    a. Systemic lupus erythematosus
    b. Rheumatoid arthritis
    c. Psoriatic arthropathy
    d. Scleroderma
    e. Mixed connective tissue disease

88. In COVID-19, serum IgM antibody secretion occurs how soon after onset of symptoms:
    a. Days 1-3
    b. Days 3-5
    c. Days 5-7
    d. Days 7-9
    e. Days 9-11

89. The most common cause of viral encephalitis is:
    a.   Enteroviruses
    b.   Varicella-zoster virus
    c.   Arboviruses
    d.   West Nile virus
    e.   Herpes simplex virus

90. The proportion of people with latent tuberculosis who will progress to active tuberculosis is:
    a.   5-10%
    b.   10-20%
    c.   20-40%
    d.   40-60%
    e.   50-90%

91. West Nile virus:
    a.   Is maintained in a human-mosquito-human cycle
    b.   Is spread only by the Aedes mosquito
    c.   Transmission is not seasonal
    d.   Neuroinvasive disease develops in 25% of those infected
    e.   Treatment is supportive

92. Hepatitis E virus:
    a.   There are four known genotypes
    b.   The majority of those infected are symptomatic
    c.   Is a DNA virus
    d.   Is a zoonotic disease
    e.   Is not transmitted via blood products

93. Which of the following is required for the diagnosis of hepatorenal syndrome with acute kidney injury (HRS-AKI):
   a. Proteinuria >500g per day
   b. Haematuria >50RBCs per high power field
   c. Normal renal ultrasound
   d. Current use of nephrotoxic drugs
   e. Absence of ascites

94. Which of the following do not increase the risk of gout:
   a. Coffee intake
   b. Obesity
   c. Fructose-sweetened drinks
   d. Dietary red meat
   e. Dietary seafood

95. Which of the following is more likely to occur in anterior circulation stroke than in posterior circulation stroke:
   a. Coma
   b. Vertigo
   c. Dysphasia
   d. Diplopia
   e. Ataxia

96. Fabry disease is a lysosomal storage disease occurring due to deficiency in the enzyme:
   a. β-glucosidase
   b. Sphingomyelinase
   c. α-galactosidase A
   d. α-iduronidase
   e. Iduronate-2-sulphate

97. Fibrates act mainly to reduce:

    a.   Triglyceride levels
    b.   LDL-C levels
    c.   HDL-C levels
    d.   Total cholesterol levels
    e.   VLDL-C levels

98. The most common manifestation of erysipelothrix rhusiopathiae infection in humans is:

    a.   Endocarditis
    b.   Septic arthritis
    c.   Meningitis
    d.   Septicaemia
    e.   Erysipeloid

99. Chikungunya fever:

    a.   Most of those infected with Chikungunya virus are asymptomatic
    b.   Retro-orbital headache is a diagnostic feature
    c.   Mortality rate is 50% for those infected
    d.   May present years after an insect b te
    e.   Arthralgia may persist for years after infection

100. Idiosyncratic drug-induced liver injury:

    a.   Is most commonly cause by paracetamol
    b.   Is a diagnosis of exclusion
    c.   Will not cause cholestasis
    d.   Is rarely fatal
    e.   Rechallenge with the drug is always contraindicated

1. Answer e

TAVI has evolved in recent years to become an alternative to surgical aortic valve replacement in selected patients with aortic stenosis. At present it is primarily used to those with a high operative risk for surgical aortic valve replacement but this may change in the coming years.[6,7]

2. Answer c

The most common site for arterial thrombosis in APS is the cerebral arterial system. The most common site for venous thrombosis in APS is the deep veins of the leg.[8]

3. Answer c

Spontaneous bacterial peritonitis (SBP) is infection of the ascitic fluid without a surgical cause. It may be asymptomatic in up to a third of cases. All patients admitted with decompensated liver disease and ascites should have an ascitic tap to exclude SBP. A polymorphonuclear cell count of >250/mm^3 is diagnostic. Antibiotics should be commenced prior to culture results if SPB is suspected.[11]

4. Answer e

The proportion of duodenal ulcers associated with Helicobacter pylori is reported as 90% and the proportion of gastric ulcers associated with Helicobacter pylori is reported as 70%.[15]

5. Answer a

ACE inhibitor-induced angioedema is more common in African-Americans, women and smokers. It usually occurs in the first week after starting treatment but may occur later, and may occur up to one month after stopping the medication. It is potentially fatal if the upper airways are involved so the medication should be stopped permanently if it occurs.[16]

6. Answer c

Erythema migrans is a spreading rash which is diagnostic of Lyme disease. Erythema migrans may appear from 3 days to 3 months after a tick bite and may last for weeks. A typical localised immune reaction to an insect bite can appear similar to erythema migrans but usually appears and resolves within 48 hours. Lyme serology may be negative in the first few weeks of infection or in the immunosuppressed. It has a seasonal occurrence

7. Answer d

Marfan syndrome is an autosomal dominant disorder involving mutations to the fibrillin 1 gene (FBN1). Although all of the complications on the above list can be associated with Marfan syndrome, aortic root disease occurs in up to 80% of affected individuals and its complications are the primary source of morbidity and mortality. Surveillance, medications such as beta blockers and surgical intervention have greatly increased the life expectancy of those with Marfan syndrome.[27,28]

8. Answer a

The maximum amount of air that can be expelled from the lungs during a forced expiration from a position of full inspiration is the forced vital capacity (FVC). The maximum amount of air that can be expelled from the lungs in the first second of a forced expiration from a position of full inspiration is the forced expiratory volume in 1 second (FEV1). The maximum amount of air which can be exhaled or inspired during a forced or slow manoeuvre can refer to the vital capacity (VC) or forced vital capacity (FVC). The average expired flow over the middle half of a forced expiratory manoeuvre is the forced expiratory flow 25-75% ($FEF_{25-75\%}$)[30]

9. Answer   a

MGUS can be divided into low-risk, intermediate-risk and high-risk. Low-risk is defined as M protein <1.5g/dl, IgG type and a normal kappa-lambda light chain ratio (0.26 to 1.65). The risk of MGUS progressing to myeloma is about 1% per year, but about half of MGUS are low-risk which only has a 5% risk of progression over 20 years and less frequent surveillance is necessary.[31]

10. Answer b

Dengue fever is caused by a single-stranded RNA virus of the Flavivirus family and is spread by Aedes mosquitoes. It is the fastest-spreading mosquito-borne viral infection. It may be asymptomatic, but severe cases can cause haemorrhagic fever. There are four serotypes of the virus and infection with one type confers lifelong immunity to that serotype only. It is thought infection with a second serotype may increase the risk of haemorrhagic fever due to an immune reaction. Most deaths occur in children and there is no vaccine or anti-viral treatment.[33]

11. Answer d

Raynaud's phenomenon usually affects the hands but may also affect the toes, nose, earlobes and nipples. The colour change sequence is white-blue-red. Secondary Raynaud's, for example due to a connective tissue disease, is more likely to lead to complications such as digital necrosis. Nailfold capillaroscopy is useful to distinguish between primary and secondary Raynaud's, with abnormal nailfold capillaroscopy pointing to secondary Raynaud's. Raynaud's may be the initial presentation of a secondary cause. Calcium channel blockers have been shown to reduce the severity and frequency of attacks.[34]

12. Answer c

Malaria is transmitted by Anopheles mosquitoes, all the others by Aedes mosquitoes.[23]

13. Answer e

Statin intolerance and discontinuation is most commonly due to statin-associated muscle symptoms (SAMS). Statin discontinuation is associated with increased cardiovascular risk when compared with those who continue treatment. The prevalence of SAMS is controversial, with some studies suggesting a 'nocebo' effect, with reproduction of SAMS in some patients taking placebo. SAMS can range from myalgia, myopathy, myosotis to myonecrosis (including rhabdomyolysis). In milder symptoms such as myalgia there may not be a CK rise. The incidence of more serious reactions such as myosotis (CKx10 upper limit of normal) is about 1 per 10000 per year and rhabdomyolysis (CKx40 upper limit of normal) about 1 per 100000 per year. Alternative statins or dosage changes can be tried, but vitamin D and coenzyme 10 supplements are not useful.[38]

14. Answer e

Spondyloarthropathies are a group of chronic inflammatory conditions with characteristic features of axial inflammation (spine and sacro-iliac joints), peripheral features (dactylitis, enthesitis, mono- or oligoarthritis) and extra-articular manifestations (uveitis, inflammatory bowel disease, psoriasis). They can be classed as predominantly axial or peripheral. Axial spondyloarthropathies are subdivided into those with radiographic changes in the sacro-iliac joints (ankylosing spondylitis) and those without (non-radiographic axial spondyloarthritis). Axial spondyloarthropathies occur equally in men and women. Not all affected individuals are positive for HLA B 27, for example 90% of those with ankylosing spondylitis are positive. An MRI scan of lumbosacral spine may miss features of ankylosing spondylitis as it may not include the sacro-iliac joints and may not include STIR-weighted images to detect bone oedema. Low back pain in axial spondyloarthropathies tends to improve with movement. The uveitis associated with spondyloarthropathies can be sight-threatening.[45,46]

15. Answer b

Monogenic disorders are conditions which are caused by mutation to a specific gene and are inherited in a Mendelian pattern as autosomal dominant, recessive or X-linked There are estimated to be over 10000 monogenic disorders.[49] Sickle cell disease is the most common monogenic disorder. It is inherited in an autosomal recessive manner, and occurs due to an amino acid substitution with valine for glutamic acid in the beta globin chain (Glu6Val, rs334].[48]

16. Answer d

Mycobacterium tuberculosis spreads via aerosol droplets so only pulmonary disease is communicable. Multi-drug resistant TB is defined as TB resistant to the two first-line drugs rifampicin and isoniazid. Latent TB present for less than 2 years is at higher risk of re-activation. Lifetime risk of latent TB reactivation is 5-10%.[54,23]

17. Answer b

Sarcoidosis may affect any part of the neurological system. In 90% of cases neurosarcoidosis sarcoid also affects other systems. The cranial nerves may be affected, most commonly cranial nerves II, VII and VIII. Optic neuritis affects visual acuity in one third of cases. Facial palsy be unilateral or bilateral and usually resolves, with 90% resolving after steroid treatment. Neurosarcoidosis nearly always requires treatment with steroids because spontaneous resolution is uncommon and permanent neurological deficits may occur. Treatment with other disease modifying drugs may be necessary as neurosarcoidosis often recurs.[61]

18. Answer a

The most common cause of right ventricular failure is left ventricular failure.[67]

19. Answer b

The McDonald criteria, originally published in 2001 and most recently updated in 2017, are used primarily to help identify multiple sclerosis in those with clinically isolated syndrome. A clinically isolated syndrome is a monophasic clinical episode with patient-reported symptoms and objective findings reflecting a focal or multifocal inflammatory demyelinating event in the CNS, developing acutely or subacutely, with a duration of at least 24 h, with or without recovery, and in the absence of fever or infection, similar to a typical multiple sclerosis relapse (attack and exacerbation) but in a patient not known to have multiple sclerosis. The criteria use clinical and MRI features to establish dissemination in space and time for inflammatory CNS lesions to diagnose multiple sclerosis. The demonstration of CSF-specific oligoclonal bands can be used to demonstrate dissemination in time in those with one clinical attack, although this does not itself establish a diagnosis. Serial MRI scans can be useful but not always needed if dissemination in space and time can be demonstrated at initial presentation.[90,91]

20. Answer d

Penicillin allergy is not always lifelong, with up to 50% resolving after five years. Cross-reactivity with cephalosporins is less likely than previously described although is more likely to occur with first generation amino-cephalosporins such as cephalexin, with cross reaction likely to be less than the 10% previously thought. A label of penicillin allergy has been associated with an increased risk of adverse outcomes such as MRSA, clostridium difficile and vancomycin-resistant enterococci infection and colonisation. True penicillin allergy is difficult to separate from a penicillin allergy label obtained after a childhood rash or other non severe adverse reactions, but it has been estimated that up to 90% of those with a label of penicillin allergy could safely take penicillins. Oral penicillin challenge can be tried after careful assessment of an individual's reported penicillin allergy history, but should always be tried in a supervised hospital setting.[95,96]

21. Answer d

Drug reaction with eosinophilia and systemic symptoms (DRESS syndrome) is an uncommon drug hypersensitivity reaction. It tends to present with widespread rash, facial oedema, fever, lymphadenopathy and variable visceral involvement. Eosinophilia usually occurs but is not universal. The liver is the most common organ involved besides the skin. Mortality is 10%. Morbilliform rash is the most common skin manifestation although urticaria, erythema multiforme or pustular rash may occur, and there may be some overlap with features of Stevens-Johnson syndrome. Given the heterogenous nature of its presentation, facial oedema is seen as a useful characteristic to help differentiate it from other severe illnesses such as sepsis.[97]

22. Answer a

Methotrexate is a very successful medication, progressing from a cytotoxic agent used in cancer treatment to a cornerstone in disease modifying treatments for many rheumatological conditions. Current regimes of low dose methotrexate minimise adverse effects although the risk persists, with gastrointestinal manifestations the most common (nausea, stomatitis, hepatotoxicity), and interstitial pneumonitis and cytopenias also among the most significant. Uncommon dermatological adverse effects include skin nodulosis and alopecia. No adverse effects on bone mineral density have been demonstrated from methotrexate use.[98]

23. Answer e

For those with atrial fibrillation stroke risk is higher in females and in those with diabetes. Heart failure is a risk factor for both reduced and preserved ejection fraction. Stroke risk is higher in valvular than non-valvular atrial fibrillation. Hypertension is also a risk factor with increased risk for higher blood pressure readings.[102]

24. Answer e

Most cases of Parkinson's disease do not have an associated family history (simplex case) but in about 15% of cases there are family members also affected (familial Parkinson's disease). 5-10% of Parkinson's disease is monogenic, that is attributable to one genetic mutation. This may be inherited in an autosomal dominant, recessive or X linked manner, with several responsible genes identified. The cumulative lifetime risk of developing Parkinson's disease is 4% in the general population but this increases to 8% in first degree relatives of cases. MRI brain is useful only in excluding other neurological conditions. Parkinson's disease most commonly presents in older individuals, but can present at an earlier age. Juvenile onset Parkinson's disease can present before 20 years of age and is usually an autosomal recessive monogenic condition, with spasticity, dystonia and dementia often present. Adult onset Parkinson's disease presents at age 20 to 50 years of age and late onset Parkinson's disease presents over the age of 50.[104]

25. Answer d

Complications of coeliac disease are more common in those with a late diagnosis of coeliac disease over the age of 50 years. 2-3% of those with coeliac disease have negative serological markers, with seronegative coeliac disease having a female predominance, higher risks of complications, associated autoimmune disease and development of refractory coeliac disease. Hyposplenism occurs in 30% of those with coeliac disease. Small bowel adenocarcinoma is a rare malignancy increasingly seen in association with coeliac disease. It remains less common than intestinal lymphoma, which usually develops in those with refractory coeliac disease (persistent malabsorption in spite of gluten free diet).[105]

26. Answer a

Glucose intolerance and diabetes mellitus are features of Cushing syndrome and not hypoglycaemia.[109,112]

27. Answer c

In early cystic fibrosis staphylococcus aureus and haemophilus influenza are prominent, but the most commonly isolated respiratory pathogen in cystic fibrosis is pseudomonas aeruginosa. Colonisation with pseudomonas aeruginosa is also one of the main predictors of morbidity and mortality in cystic fibrosis.[123]

28. Answer b

Vaughan Williams Class I anti-arrhythmics are sodium channel blockers, with flecainide in class IC. The subdivisions of class I anti-arrhythmics depend on its effect on repolarisation and 'refractoriness'. Class II are betablockers. Class III are potassium channel blockers such as amiodarone. Class IV are calcium channel blockers.[124]

29. Answer c

The relationship between LDL reduction and reduced cardiovascular risk is linear. For every reduction of 39 mg/dl (1.0 mmol/L) in LDL cholesterol level, statins confer relative reductions in cardiovascular events by 22% and in all-cause mortality by 10%. Ezetimibe increases hepatic LDL expression by reducing intestinal and biliary cholesterol absorption. Its role at present is mainly as add-on in high risk patients where intensive statin therapy is insufficient. Long-chain n–3 polyunsaturated fatty acids such as eicosapentaenoic acid (EPA) and docosahexaenoic acid have not been shown to reduce cardiovascular events and mortality, despite their positive effects in triglyceride reduction. Icosapent ethyl, a highly purified form of EPA has shown promise in reducing cardiovascular events. PCSK9 inhibitors are injectable monoclonal antibodies which inhibit internal degradation of LDL receptors, and lead to a marked reduction in LDL. Studies have shown a relative risk reduction of 15% in cardiovascular events and they are currently finding a role in high risk patients where statins and ezetimibe are not tolerated or are not sufficient in reducing LDL.[127]

30. Answer b

Hodgkin's lymphoma is a malignancy arising from germinal centre and post-germinal centre B cells. It is characterised by the presence of multinucleate giant cells or large mononuclear cells known as Hodgkin and Reed Sternberg (HRS) cells. Painless enlarging lymphadenopathy is a common presentation of Hodgkins lymphoma. The most common sites are mediastinum and left or right side of neck. Other sites include splenic, axillary, abdominal, hilar or inguinofemoral in descending order of frequency.[129,130]

31. Answer a

Risk factors for recurrence in an individual with DVT or PE include proximal DVT, unprovoked DVT or PE, active malignancy, underlying hypercoagulable state, post thrombotic syndrome, raised BMI and advanced age. Residual venous thrombosis and elevated D Dimers after discontinuation of anticoagulation may also be risk factors. Patients with unprovoked VTE have a risk of recurrence reported to be between 25% and 30% at 5 to 10 years after the initial event. These risk factors are used to decide on duration and anticoagulation in venous thromboembolic disease.[136]

32. Answer c

Filoviruses include the Ebola virus and Marburg virus species. They are filamentous RNA viruses. They are zoonotic pathogens and they are maintained in animal reservoirs. They can be transmitted to humans causing outbreaks from time to time. The infections they cause can have a high mortality rate. Spread occurs most commonly via mucous membranes but may occur via the percutaneous route occasionally.[138]

33. Answer e

Loop diuretics are useful in HFpEF to improve symptoms and quality of life but do not improve mortality or reduce hospitalisations. In contrast to heart failure with low ejection fraction <40%, medications have not been shown to reduce endpoints such as mortality in HFpEF.[139]

34. Answer e

Fournier's gangrene is a necrotising fasciitis of the perineal, perianal and genital areas. It tends to occur from a small nidus of infection which rapidly spreads to cause a fulminant necrotising fasciitis and can progress quickly to sepsis and multiorgan failure. It is more common in those with certain vulnerabilities such as diabetes, immunosuppression or alcoholism. It is an emergency and early surgical debridement has been shown to reduce the high mortality. It is more common in men but can occur in women. Previously most cases were idiopathic but it is now recognised as being caused by multiple pathogens acting synergistically, most commonly Escherichia coli, Klebsiella pneumonia, Bacteroides fragilis, Staphylococcus aureus and sometimes fungal pathogens.[140,141]

35. Answer e

Intestinal inflammation in ulcerative colitis usually begins in the rectum and extends proximally in a continuous, circumferential pattern. Rectal sparing may occur due to topical or systemic medications and should not necessarily be seen as evidence of Crohn's disease.[142]

36. Answer b

Infective endocarditis (IE) is a multisystem disease arising from infection of the endocardium of the heart. The average age of those affected has increased due to the reduced incidence of rheumatic heart disease and its role in IE, as well as an ageing population more prone to degenerative valvular disease, increasing use of valvular surgery and implantable cardiac devices. Bacteraemia is a pre-requisite for development of IE. The normal endocardium is resistant to bacterial colonisation but a process of platelet-fibrin aggregation on damaged valves and endocardium can lead to vegetation formation. Gram positive bacteria such as staphylococcus and streptococcus remain the most common causative pathogens. 50% will develop positive rheumatoid factors after 6 weeks, and levels decrease with antibiotic treatment. Antibiotic prophylaxis started being used in the 1930s after it was discovered that dental extraction may be a risk for IE in those with a history of rheumatic fever. In more recent years its use has been rationalised, with some countries phasing out its use, and others recommending its use only in high risk individuals.[143,144]

37. Answer c

Transient ischaemic attack (TIA) involves transient neurological signs or symptoms usually lasting seconds to minutes and usually less than one hour, with no radiological signs of an acute ischaemic infarct on brain radiology. Transient ischaemic attack (TIA) symptoms are likely to be motor, sensory (for example motor or sensory deficit in two limbs or one limb and the face) or visual (monocular blindness or homonymous hemianopia), or involve speech disturbance such as aphasia or dysarthria. Transient loss of consciousness is much less likely to be cause by a TIA.[150]

38. Answer b

The specificity of a test refers to the proportion of people without a condition who have a negative test result. It can be calculated as:

true negatives/(false positives + true negatives).

The proportion of people with a condition who have a positive test result is the sensitivity of a test.

The proportion of people with a condition who have a negative test result is the false negative rate.

The proportion of people without a condition who have a positive test result is the false positive rate.

The proportion of people with a condition with a given test result (either positive or negative) divided by the proportion of people without the condition with that result is the likelihood ratio.[151]

39. Answer b

Hypersensitivity pneumonitis is a delayed allergic reaction to external agents leading to inflammation of the alveoli, terminal bronchioles and alveolar interstitium. It can present acutely with cough, fever and dyspnoea, or as chronic disease, with progressive pulmonary fibrosis which is not reversible. It can be a type 3 hypersensitivity reaction (immune complex mediated, more important in the acute form) or type 4 hypersensitivity reaction (T lymphocyte mediated, more important in the chronic form). In the subacute phase histological analysis of lung biopsy will show interstitial lymphoplastic pneumonitis, non-necrotising granulomas or giant cells and cellular bronchiolitis. Corticosteroids are first line in treatment of acute and subacute disease, but have not been shown to influence progression, and emphasis should be on identifying and removing the causative agent. Farmer's lung (Aspergillus species) and bird fancier's lung (Avian proteins in droppings and on feathers) are the most commonly identified forms and may affect children.[156,157]

40. Answer b

Acitretin is a retinoid used in the treatment of psoriasis. All of these are known side effects, but cheilitis is the most common, occurring dose dependently in all patients.[158]

41. Answer b

Teriparatide is a truncated parathyroid hormone analogue. Parathyroid hormone causes marked bone loss, but intermittent parathyroid hormone exposure is associated with net bone formation. This finding led to the development of teriparatide which has been shown to reduce the risk of vertebral fractures by 65% and non-vertebral fractures by 53%. It has been associated with an increased risk of osteosarcoma in rodents which led to its licencing being limited to two years. No association with osteosarcoma has been found in humans.[160]

42. Answer d

In chronic hepatitis C infection 10-20% will develop cirrhosis over 20-30 years of infection. Antibody testing cannot distinguish between acute and chronic infection. Antibodies will also persist in individuals who have spontaneously cleared the virus or who have had successful treatment. Antibodies do not confer immunity from future infection. Those who have a positive antibody test should also have a HCV RNA test, which is specific for active infection. The presence of a positive antibody test with HCV RNA viral load greater than the level of detection have an active hepatitis C infection. Transmission is usually by percutaneous spread such as intravenous drug use, via blood products or vertical transmission during childbirth, with sexual transmission less common.[162,163]

43. Answer a

Rheumatoid factor antibodies are pentameric IgM antibodies that bind to the Fc portion of human IgG.[164,165]

44. Answer a

Common variable immunodeficiency is characterised by hypogammaglobulinemia and recurrent infections. B cell levels are usually normal suggesting an abnormality in their differentiation to plasma cells. They are a heterogenous group of disorders, many of which are of unknown cause. Known monogenic mutations account for less than 20% of cases. Respiratory infections are the most common type of recurrent infection with bronchiectasis and interstitial lung disease occurring as a result. Gastrointestinal infections are also common causing acute or chronic diarrhoea, especially in those with undetectable IgA levels which tend not to improve with immunoglobulin treatment. Helicobacter infection does not appear to be increased, possibly due to antibiotic treatments for other infections. There is increased risk of malignancy and associated autoimmune disorders, thought to be due to disordered immunoregulatory factors.[171,174]

45. Answer b

The most common chromosomal condition associated with intellectual disability is Down syndrome or trisomy 21.[175]

46. Answer a

Thrombophilias are inherited or acquired blood conditions that increase the propensity for vascular thrombosis. The most common inherited thrombophilias are Factor V Leiden and prothrombin gene FII G20210A polymorphism (PGM). Deficiencies in protein C, protein S and antithrombin are less common inherited thrombophilias. The most common acquired thrombophilia is antiphospholipid syndrome, and others include Bechet's disease and myeloproliferative disorders. Acquired thrombophilias are more likely to cause arterial thrombosis than inherited thrombophilias, which tend to cause venous thromboembolic disease only. Testing for protein C, protein S and antithrombin deficiencies are often unreliable during an acute thromboembolic event as levels are likely to be decreased, but Factor V Leiden and PGM can be tested anytime. Routine testing for thrombophilia is not necessary in most patients with venous thromboembolic (VTE) disease , as the risk of recurring VTE is uncertain in many thrombophilias so the results will not change management. The decision regarding duration of anticoagulation in VTE should be made depending on whether the incident was provoked or unprovoked, bleeding risk and family history.

Inherited thrombophilias are relatively common in the Caucasian population and much less common in non-white individuals.[179]

47. Answer a

Porphyrias consist of nine conditions characterised by alterations in enzymes involved in heme biosynthesis. Acute intermittent porphyria (AIP) is the most common acute form, and is characterised by potentially life-threatening acute attacks most commonly causing abdominal pain, nausea, hypertension, tachycardia, anxiety and agitation. Neurological manifestation may progress to confusion, convulsions and respiratory paralysis. Peripheral neuropathy is also a feature. Skin manifestations are uncommon in AIP. Dark or reddish urine may be observed which may darken further after exposure to light. It is inherited as an autosomal dominant trait and occurs due to mutations affecting the production of porphobilinogen deaminase (PBGD) an enzyme involved in heme synthesis. Most heterozygotes will never have an acute attack, as enzyme production is sufficient from the unaffected gene. Acute attacks can be triggered by certain medications such as exogenous oestrogens, barbiturates, rifampicin. Fasting and alcohol can also trigger attacks.[181]

48. Answer e

Hyperthyroidism is a state of increased production and secretion of thyroid hormone from the thyroid gland. Thyrotoxicosis is a clinical syndrome of excess circulating thyroid hormone of any cause. Excess thyroid hormone intake is a cause of thyrotoxicosis and not hyperthyroidism. Hyperthyroidism is more likely to occur in iodine deficient areas and incidence decreases after introduction of salt iodisation programmes. The incidence of hyperthyroidism increases with age and is more common in women.

Graves' disease is the most common cause of hyperthyroidism in iodine sufficient areas, but toxic multinodular goitre or solitary toxic adenoma may cause 50% of cases in iodine deficient areas.[188]

49. Answer c

Primary aldosteronism occurs due to excess aldosterone levels in spite of a sodium and volume avid state where renin and angiotensin II levels are suppressed. It is the most common cause of secondary hypertension and is likely to be underdiagnosed with a significant group affected subclinically. It increases mortality through effects on the cardiovascular and renal systems, as well as other effects such as a link with obstructive sleep apnoea. It may cause refractory hypertension. Opinions vary as regards who should be screened, with some experts advocating screening in all people with hypertension. A high ratio of aldosterone to renin has been shown to be an effective screening tool, although the cut-off level required to progress to more dynamic testing is not agreed. Dynamic testing involves one of an oral or intravenous sodium challenge, a captopril challenge test or fludrocortisone challenge test. Failure to suppress aldosterone levels in one of these tests indicates primary aldosteronism. Radiological work up is important, to differentiate between unilateral and bilateral causes as well as to look for signs of a malignant renal carcinoma (benign adenomas are usually <2cm, carcinoma usually >6cm). Unilateral and bilateral causes are managed differently. Unilateral causes such as a functioning adenoma can be managed surgically. Cases not amenable to surgery can be managed with mineralocorticoid receptor antagonists such as spironolactone or eplerenone.

Although most adrenal incidentalomas are non-functioning, all should be screened for primary aldosteronism.[192,193]

50. Answer e

Hereditary haemorrhagic telangiectasia (HHT) is an autosomal dominant condition caused by genetic mutations affecting angiogenesis resulting in telangiectasia and arteriovenous malformations (AVMs). Two genetic mutations (ENG gene coding for endoglin protein and ANVRL1 gene encoding for the ALK1 protein) account for 95% of cases. All types of mutation have been reported: missense, nonsense, deletions, insertions and splice site. Affected family members usually have unique mutations of the affected genes, and level of severity can vary between members of the same family. Epistaxis is the most common symptom. Heritable pulmonary arterial hypertension may be associated with HHT due to shunting through pulmonary AVMs but it is rare. Telangiectasias arise due to post capillary venous dilatation.[204]

51. Answer e

Wilson's disease is an autosomal recessive disease involving abnormalities in copper metabolism. It is universally fatal without treatment. It occurs due to mutation to the ATP7B gene which encodes a transmembrane copper-transporting ATPase leading to accumulation of copper in various organs. The liver is the organ most commonly affected, reflecting its central role in copper homeostasis. After the liver, the neurological system is most commonly affected. Diagnosis can be difficult. Serum ceruloplasmin levels may by in the low-normal range in 50% of those with active liver disease, and diagnosis may depend on a combination of serum and urinary copper, serum ceruloplasmin measurement, measurement of hepatic copper content and mutational analysis. Liver biopsy in the initial stages shows changes indistinguishable from non-alcoholic fatty liver, progressing to cirrhosis in later stages. There is a large variety in disease severity, possibly reflecting the type of mutation or epigenetic and environmental factors. The most severe form, acute liver failure due to Wilson's disease, occurs predominantly in young females.[208]

52. Answer b

Osmotic demyelination syndrome (ODS) (formerly known as central pontine myelinolysis) occurs due to overly rapid correction of chronic hypotonic hyponatraemia. Serum sodium concentration is the main determinant of serum osmolality and the reduction in osmolality in hyponatraemia leads to adaptations in the brain which reduce the risk of cerebral oedema. These adaptations cause the brain to be vulnerable to ODS. Individuals with alcohol dependence, hypokalaemia, malnutrition and advanced liver disease are more vulnerable to ODS.[210]

53. Answer c

Chest x-ray is not indicated in all patients with COVID-19 as many patients will have mild illness not requiring hospital referral. Recommendations vary regarding indications for performing chest x-ray in COVID-19, but it is usually performed where COVID-19 pneumonia is clinically suspected. Typical findings on chest X-ray are ground glass opacities and horizontal linear opacities affecting the peripheral and lower zones, progressing to white-out of the lung fields in more severe cases. However these are not specific changes and are seen in many other conditions. Chest x ray may be normal in COVID-19 pneumonia.[212]

54. Answer b

Polymyalgia rheumatica (PMR) is the second most common inflammatory disease in the elderly (after rheumatoid arthritis) and is characterised by pain and stiffness of the shoulder and hip girdles. 20% of patients with PMR will have associated giant cell arteritis, while 40-60% of patients with giant cell arteritis will have PMR. Diagnosis is made using a scoring system in those with new onset symptoms and raised inflammatory markers, using clinical symptoms, absence of rheumatoid factor and joint ultrasound findings. The presence of subdeltoid bursitis, biceps tenosynovitis, glenohumeral synovitis, hip synovitis or trochanteric bursitis on joint ultrasound are suggestive of a positive diagnosis.[219,220,221]

55. Answer c

The Beighton score is used to assess joint hypermobility and consists of five clinical manoeuvres:
- Passive dorsiflexion of the 5th finger more than 90 degrees
- Passive flexion of the thumb to the forearm
- Hyperextension of the elbow to more than 10 degrees

- Hyperextension of the knee to more than 10 degrees
- Forward flexion of the trunk with knees fully extended and palms resting on the floor

1 point is attributable for the first four criteria if uniliateral and 2 points if bilateral, and one point if the fifth criteria is fulfilled. Joint hypermobility may be localised to one or two joints or may be generalised, with a score of at least 5 to diagnose generalised joint hypermobility.

The Beighton score is used to assess of joint hypermobility syndrome (JHS) and hypermobile Ehlers Danlos syndrome in the Brighton criteria and Villefranche criteria respectively. JHS refers to generalised joint hypermobility plus chronic musculoskeletal pain.[223]

56. Answer e

Trigeminal neuralgia is characterised by severe short spasms of pain occurring the in the distribution of one or more branches of the trigeminal nerve. Incidence increases with advancing age. The pain is often triggered by an innocuous stimulus such as a breeze or light touch to the face, and the location of pain may not correspond to the location of the stimulus. Pain will only affect the areas of sensory distribution of the trigeminal nerve. Pain in the area overlying the angle of the mandible, outer ear (excepting the tragus) and posterior third of the scalp are not supplied by the trigeminal nerve so pain in these areas indicates another diagnosis.

Trigeminal neuralgia may be classical, secondary or idiopathic. Classical is the most common and is caused by intracranial vascular compression of the trigeminal nerve root. Secondary trigeminal neuralgia occurs in 15% of cases and is due an underlying neurological cause such as multiple sclerosis or a benign cerebellopontine angle tumour.[224]

57. Answer a

Thyroid nodules are common and often detected incidentally on radiology performed for another reason. All patients with an incidentally detected thyroid nodule should have a dedicated ultrasound to assess the thyroid gland and neck. Features suggestive of a malignant nodule are microcalcifications, hypoechogenicity of the nodule compared with the surrounding gland parenchyma, irregular margins and shape taller than wide on transverse view.

Most malignant nodules are solid, so cystic or spongiform appearance of suggest a benign nodule. These features are not absolute and thyroid nodules should be managed by a specialist.[228,229]

58. Answer e

QT interval is measured from the beginning of the QRS complex to the end of the T wave.[232,233]

59. Answer d

Clostridium difficile, a gram positive, anaerobic, spore-forming, toxin producing bacillus, was officially renamed Clostridioides difficile in 2016, to reflect differences between this species and other members of the clostridium genus. It has been known as a gut commensal for many years, and its association with diarrhoeal infection has increased since the introduction of antibiotics.[244]

60. Answer e

Upper extremity deep vein thrombosis (UEDVT) accounts for 5% of all deep vein thrombosis. It may be primary or secondary. Primary UEDVT is usually associated with anatomical abnormalities causing venous compression as well as strenuous upper limb muscular effort. Secondary UEDVT is most commonly associated with malignancy or indwelling lines. Inherited or acquired thrombophilias may be present but are a less important cause. Complications include pulmonary embolus and post-thrombotic syndrome of the arm.[245]

61. Answer c

Typical Alzheimer's disease is the most common presentation of dementia in those over 65 years of age. It is most commonly associated with medial temporal or parietal lobe atrophy on brain imaging and a positive amyloid PET scan.

Atypical presentations of Alzheimer's disease may occur under the age of 65 years. Visual spatial, attention, executive or language skills may be more affected. These cases may have atypical features also on brain imaging.[247]

62. Answer c

'Non-valvular' atrial fibrillation refers to atrial fibrillation in somebody who does not have moderate to severe mitral stenosis or mechanical heart valves.[248]

63. Answer c

Differentiating type 1 from type 2 diabetes in adults can be quite difficult as 40% of new cases of type 1 diabetes occur in patients over the age of 30 years.

Anti-glutamic acid decarboxylase autoantibodies (anti-GAD) are the most sensitive autoantibody test for the diagnosis of type 1 diabetes and are present in 84% of patients with type 1 diabetes.

Insulin autoantibodies (IAA) are dependent on age and sex, and are present in 81% of children under 10 years of age with type 1 diabetes as against 61% in older patients. There is a male:female ratio in adults of 2:1.

Insulinoma-associated 2 autoantibodies (IA2) are present in 58% of patients with type 1 diabetes.

Islet cell cytoplasmic autoantibodies (ICA) are present in 70-80% of patients with new onset type 1 diabetes.

Zinc transporter 8 autoantibodies (ZnT8Ab) are present in 80% of patients with type 1 diabetes with a very high specificity of 99%.[273]

64. Answer e

Sjogren's syndrome is characterised by dry mouth and eyes (keratoconjunctivitis sicca) and a variety of extraglandular features. It may be primary or secondary to another chronic inflammatory disease such as SLE or rheumatoid arthritis. Anti-Ro antibodies are found in 60% and anti-La antibodies are found in 40%. Rheumatoid factor is positive in 80% of cases.

Salivary gland biopsy can be helpful in diagnosis demonstrated lack of salivary secretion. Genital dryness can cause dyspareunia. There is increased incidence of developing non-Hodgkin B cell lymphoma.[265]

65. Answer d

Herpes zoster (shingles) occurs due to reactivation of latent varicella zoster virus. It may affect a single dermatome, overlapping dermatomes or may be disseminated. It can recur especially in the immunocompromised. Rash may be preceded by neuropathic pain. In zoster sine herpete pain is evident without occurrence of rash. Visceral zoster may affect internal organs with pancreatitis, hepatitis and gastritis described. Encephalitis, meningitis and myelitis may occur with possible long term neurological sequelae.[249]

66. Answer d

Todd paralysis is a transient, localised and functional paralysis occurring after a focal seizure. It may last minutes to hours and its duration reflects seizure duration. It is of value in lateralising the hemisphere of seizure origin and is the hallmark of a focal seizure.[259]

67. Answer c

Dementia with Lewy bodies (DLB) refers to a syndrome arising from intraneuronal deposition of Lewy bodies within the cortex and substantia nigra. It is distinguished from Parkinson's disease with dementia (PDD) by restricting the diagnosis of DLB to those with dementia preceding or within one year of diagnosis of parkinsonism. Some experts believe that DLB and PDD are part of the same syndrome.

Central features required for a diagnosis of DLB include spontaneous features of parkinsonism, pronounced fluctuations in attention and alertness and visual hallucinations (often of animals, insects, children or small people). Other features include extreme neuroleptic sensitivity, rapid eye movement sleep behaviour disorder, hypotension and depression among others.

First line of treatment is with rivastigmine patch, a cholinesterase inhibitor, which can help behavioural features of DLB prior to initiation of levodopa treatment.[247]

68. Answer a

There are two main types of autoimmune blistering disease: pemphigus and pemphigoid. Pemphigus occurs due to blistering in the epidermis and pemphigoid due to subepidermal blistering.

Pemphigus occurs due to autoantibodies targeting desmoglein 1 and desmoglein 3 (Dsg 1 and Dsg 3) which play a role in desmosomes essential for cell to cell adhesion.

Pemphigoid occurs due to autoantibodies that target components of hemidesmosomes in the basement membrane zone.[250,251,252]

69. Answer c

Inhaled corticosteroids have fallen behind long acting beta agonists (LABA) and long acting muscarinic antagonists (LAMA) in treatment guidelines for COPD. They remain indicated in particular where there are signs of asthma overlap such as a previous history of asthma or evidence of reversibility on lung function testing. They are also shown to reduce exacerbations when added to LAMA/LABA treatment but with an increase in pneumonia risk. They do not improve mortality and it does not matter if they are given in a combination inhaler or separately.[256]

70. Answer b

Scleroderma is a connective tissue disease characterised by micro vascular damage and excessive deposition of collagen in the skin and internal organs. It is divided into a localised form (morphoea) which affects the skin only, and a generalised form known as systemic sclerosis. Systemic sclerosis is further subdivided into limited cutaneous systemic scleroderma (lcSSc or CREST syndrome) and diffuse cutaneous systemic scleroderma (dcSSc). These have separate clinical features and are associated with different serological positivity. CREST syndrome is associated with positive anticentromere antibodies and dcSSc is associated with positive antipoisomerase and anti-RNAP III antibodies. Several environmental exposures are associated with scleroderma, in particular silica but not asbestos. Skin biopsy is not usually required for diagnosis.[266]

71. Answer e

Wells criteria for DVT allocates points for the following:

- Active cancer palliation or treatment in the past 6 months

- Bedridden for more than 3 days or major surgery in the past 12 weeks

- Calf swelling 3cm more than other leg

- Collateral non varicose superficial veins present

- Entire leg swollen

- Focal tenderness along the deep venous system

- Pitting oedema confined to symptomatic leg

- Paralysis, paresis or recent immobilisation of affected leg

- Previously documented DVT

All these are worth one point, with two points deducted if an alternative diagnosis is more likely.

A Wells score of 2 or more should be referred for ultrasound. A Wells score of less than 2 combined with negative D Dimers indicates a very low probability of DVT.[255]

72. Answer a

Autoimmune hepatitis is a chronic progressive liver disease characterised by high IgG levels, circulating autoantibodies, histological signs of hepatitis and a favourable response to immunosuppressive treatments. It is more common on women but does occur in men. Diagnosis can be difficult as antibodies such as ANA and smooth muscle antibodies may not be present. There may be overlap with other chronic liver disease such as primary biliary cirrhosis. Untreated disease has a poor prognosis with 5 and 10 year survival of 50% and 10% respectively. Disease severity is not necessarily reflected by higher transaminase levels, and although IgG levels are usually high, normal levels do not exclude the diagnosis.[257]

73. Answer e

Familial hypercholesterolaemia is a common inherited condition resulting in prolonged exposure to high LDL levels and premature cardiovascular disease in men and women. In its most common form t is a monogenic autosomal dominant disorder affecting LDL receptors and therefor LDL uptake from the peripheral circulation.[259]

74. Answer e

Focal motor seizures occur due to an epileptogenic lesion on the contralateral frontal lobe. Typically consciousness is not impaired. The seizure may take various forms.

Tonic contractions in one hand progressing to clonic movements in the affected area, then with spread to the ipsilateral arm and to the ipsilateral foot and leg is known as a 'Jacksonian March'. It describes the seizure activity 'marching' from one affected area to other areas on the same side of the body.

Clonic seizures involve repeated short contractions of various muscle groups lasting less than 1 to 2 seconds, and are usually brief lasting 1 to 2 minutes.

Tonic seizures consist of sustained contractions of various muscle groups lasting more than 5 to 10 seconds resulting in posturing of the limbs and whole body.

Versive seizures involve sustained, forceful, involuntary turning of the head and eyes to one side due to tonic contraction of the head and eye muscles.[259]

75. Answer c

High resolution CT scan of the lungs is the most useful investigation in diagnosis of pulmonary fibrosis. Typical features are reticulation, architectural distortion and lung volume loss. The other investigations listed may be useful to exclude other diagnoses or to elucidate a cause for lung fibrosis.[260]

76. Answer a

Darier disease is a rare autosomal dominant condition also known as keratosis follicularis. It is caused by a mutation in the ATP2A2 gene which encodes a calcium pump in the endoplasmic reticulum. This leads to aberrant junctional protein processing and poor cohesion between keratinocytes. Hyperkeratotic plaques develop in the seborrheic and intertriginous areas. Secondary infection is common. Friction, heat, sweat and sun exposure can exacerbate the disease. The oral mucosa is involved in 50% of patients.[261]

77. Answer d

Complex regional pain syndrome (CRPS) is a chronic neurological condition occurring due to a traumatic insult. It can be divided into two categories: CRPS I (previously known as reflex sympathetic dystrophy) where there is no identifiable nerve injury, and CRPS II (previously known as causalgia) where there is an identifiable nerve injury. Clinical features include changes in skin temperature and colour, oedema, hyperalgesia and allodynia, with clinical features not occurring in a dermatomal distribution. Fractures of the upper limb are the injuries most vulnerable to CRPS and distal fractures are more vulnerable than proximal fractures.[263]

78. Answer a

Benign paroxysmal positional vertigo is characterised by sudden, transitory vertigo sensation provoked by positional changes of the head with accompanying nystagmus. It is caused by aberrant signalling from the semicircular canals creating an illusion of motion. It is the most frequent cause of vertigo.[263]

79. Answer e

Mixed connective tissue disease (MCTD) refers to a rheumatological overlap syndrome with clinical features of SLE, systemic sclerosis, polymyositis and rheumatoid arthritis. It is associated with a high titre and anti-nuclear antibodies and anti-U1RNP antibodies, with other autoantibodies usually negative. The different features tend to present sequentially rather than simultaneously. Arthralgia (90%) is more common than arthritis (70%) with inflammatory muscle disease typical of myositis, Raynaud's phenomenon and sicca symptoms also common features. Lung involvement occurs in 75% with interstitial lung disease in 50% and pulmonary hypertension the most common disease related cause of death.[264]

80. Answer c

Guillain Barre syndrome is a progressive motor weakness, usually symmetrical and beginning in the legs, and reaching its maximum weakness within four weeks of onset. It is assumed to be due to an immunological response to triggers such as surgery or infection. Campylobacter jejuni infection leads to GBS in 1 in 1000 cases. The most common presentation is bilateral symmetrical motor weakness beginning in the distal lower limbs. However sensory symptoms may occur such as paraesthesia and numbness. Pain is a common and often early feature. Cranial nerves may be affected in the Miller Fischer variant. The sural nerve should be avoided in nerve conduction testing as it is often normal in GBS.[267,268]

81. Answer e

Autosomal dominant polycystic kidney disease (ADPKD) is a relatively common cause of end-stage renal disease. It is a monogenic cilia-related disorder. 80% of cases are caused by mutations in PKD1 (chromosome 16p13.3) and 15% of cases caused by mutations in FKD2 (chromosome 4q22.1) and the remainder genetically unresolved or due to rare mutations. It has a much more severe course in men although it is not clear why. The phenotype can be quite variable with some genetically affected patients developing few renal cysts. 75% of patients will progress to end-stage renal disease. 10-15% of those affected have no family history suggesting relatively common de-novo mutations. Early onset hypertension is a common feature and studies have shown the presence of hypertension in 20% or more of genetically affected children.[270]

82. Answer b

Von Willebrand's disease is the most common inherited bleeding disorder. It is characterised by mucosal bleeding and bleeding after surgery or trauma (although other types of bleeding also occur) and laboratory evidence of von Willebrand factor abnormalities. Factor VIII activity is often but not always reduced. There are three types of von Willebrand's disease. Type 1 accounts for 80% of cases and is caused by a quantitative deficiency of von Willebrand factor. Type 2 accounts for about 20% of cases and is characterised by dysfunctional von Willebrand factor. Type 3 is rare and is the most severe form, caused by complete absence of circulating von Willebrand factor. Most cases are autosomal dominant.

Diagnosis is made based on history and family history of bleeding, as well as a combination of von Willebrand factor antigen measurement, level of von Willebrand factor-dependent platelet adhesion and the coagulant activity of factor VIII. Diagnosis of the different types can be difficult, and there is controversy over what level of von Willebrand factor antigen cut-off should determine deficiency. Levels <5IU/dl are seen in type 3 disease but generally levels <30IU/dl are considered deficient. Levels of 30 to 50 IU/dl are labelled 'possible type 1 von Willebrand disease'.

Von Willebrand levels may be normal in type 2 disease, and also in type 1 disease in older people, as levels increase with age.[271]

83. Answer a

Mosaicism refers to the presence of different genotypes in one individual. It may arise by a number of mechanisms such as chromosome non-dysjunction, mutations arising during development and gene editing.[272]

84. Answer a

The World Health Organisation and America Diabetes Association criteria for diagnosis of all types of diabetes mellitus are:

Fasting plasma glucose greater than or equal to 7.0 mmol/L (126mg/dL), or

2 hour plasma glucose of greater than or equal to 11.1mmol/L (200mg/dL) during an oral glucose tolerance test using a 75g glucose load, or

HbA1c greater than or equal to 6.5% (48mmol/mol), or

Random plasma glucose of greater than or equal to 11.1mmol/L (200mg/dL) in a symptomatic patient with classic hyperglycaemia symptoms

Where a state of hyperglycaemia is uncertain, two abnormal tests are required for diagnosis.

Differentiating type 1 from type 2 diabetes in adults can be quite difficult as 40% of new cases of type 1 diabetes occur in patients over the age of 30 years.

HbA1c is not an appropriate test for diagnosing type 1 diabetes as the onset of hyperglycaemia may occur rapidly and may not be reflected in the result, and also there can be a delay in processing the test when compared to blood glucose levels.[273]

85. Answer b

Calciphylaxis is a rare life-threatening syndrome with very painful necrotic skin lesions resulting from calcific occlusion of arterioles in the skin and subcutaneous tissues. It is associated with early or end-stage renal disease, acute renal disease and those who have received a kidney transplant, but may occur rarely in those with normal renal function. It is also known as calcific uremic arteriolopathy. The lesion are very painful and become necrotic, and once the condition develops prognosis is poor, with a 6 month survival rate in ulcerated lesions of 20%.[274]

86. Answer b

Chronic kidney disease (CKD) is defined as a glomerular filtration rate (GFR) of <60ml/min of the presence of kidney damage for three months or more. Kidney damage can refer to pathological abnormalities documented by biopsy or imaging, protein-to-creatinine ratio of >200mg/g or albumin-to-creatinine ratio of >30mg/g, genetic renal disorder or h story of renal transplantation.

A rise in creatinine may be consistent with chronic kidney disease, but without duration established could also be caused by an episode of reversible acute kidney injury.[275,276]

87. Answer b

Caplan's syndrome is the presence of rheumatoid arthritis in association with a pneumoconiosis. It can be associated with exposure to coal, asbestos and/or silica. There is a separate association between silicosis and connective tissue disorders such as scleroderma.[278]

88. Answer c

In COVID-19, serum IgM and IgA antibodies are secreted by days 5 to 7 after the onset of symptoms. IgG is secreted by days 7 to 10 after onset of symptoms.[279]

89. Answer e

In many cases of encephalitis a cause is not identified. Of viral causes, 50-75% of cases (at least in the USA) are caused by herpes simplex virus. Most of the remainder are caused by varicella-zoster viruses, enteroviruses and arboviruses.[280]

90. Answer a

The proportion of people with latent tuberculosis who will progress to active tuberculosis is 5-10%.[281,282,283]

91. Answer e

West Nile virus is a flavivirus spread by mosquitoes. It is maintained in a bird-mosquito-bird cycle with humans a dead-end host. It has been detected in many bird and mosquito species but is predominantly spread by a few Culex mosquito species in North America. Outbreaks are seasonal and warm weather promotes transmission. 25% of those infected develop West Nile fever with a large variation in illness severity. <1% will develop neuroinvasive disease and this has a mortality rate of 10%. No treatment or vaccine exists.[284,285]

92. Answer d

Hepatitis E is an RNA virus and is a common infective agent worldwide. There are 8 known genotypes. The majority of infections are asymptomatic, but hepatitis E can cause acute or acute-on-chronic liver failure. Although all are thought to have the capacity to infect humans, genotypes 1-4 have been associated with most frequent human infection. Genotypes 1 and 2 are transmitted by contaminated drinking water and cause millions of infections annually in the tropics. Genotypes 3 and 4 are zoonoses and are transmitted by contaminated pork products. Blood product transmission of hepatitis E virus has been described.[286]

93. Answer c

Hepatorenal syndrome is renal impairment in those with liver cirrhosis, characterised by a reduction in renal blood flow and glomerular filtration rate.

Hepatorenal syndrome is subdivided into hepatorenal syndrome with acute kidney injury (HRS-AKI) and hepatorenal syndrome with non-acute kidney injury (HRS-NAKI). Diagnosis of HRS-AKI requires deterioration of serum creatinine to a given level within 48 hours and the absence of structural kidney injury reflected in the absence of proteinuria, haematuria and normal renal ultrasound. The criteria for diagnosis of HRS-AKI are:

Increase in serum creatinine of greater than or equal to 0.3g/dL (26.5μmol/L) within 48 hours

OR

Increase in serum creatinine greater than or equal to 1.5 times from baseline

No response to diuretic withdrawal and two day fluid challenge

Cirrhosis with ascites

Absence of shock

No current or recent use of nephrotoxic drugs

No signs of structural kidney disease

Hypovolaemia may occur in liver cirrhosis due to a number of factors, leading to acute tubular necrosis, and differentiating this from HRS-AKI can be challenging.[287]

94. Answer a

Risk factors for gout include male gender, ethnicity (more common in Afro-Caribbean, South Pacific Islanders), obesity, hypertension, renal impairment and insulin resistance, as well as diuretic use. Excess consumption of beer or spirits, red meat, seafood, fruit juices and fructose-sweetened beverages also increase risk. Fructose is the only carbohydrate that increases uric acid levels by increasing ATP degradation and insulin resistance.

Regular consumption of coffee, yogurt and vitamin C have been shown to reduce serum uric acid and risk of gout.[288]

95. Answer c

Posterior circulation stroke occurs due to occlusion of part of the vertebrobasilar arterial system affecting areas of the brain such as the brain stem, cerebellum, midbrain, thalamuses and occipital cortex. Anterior circulation stroke affects the carotid artery and branches including the anterior and middle cerebral arteries and their branches.

Coma is uncommon in anterior circulation stroke unless there is a mass effect causing raised intracranial pressure. Coma may be an acute presentation (2%) in posterior circulation stroke due to thalamic and brainstem ischaemia.

In practice the clinical presentations of posterior and anterior circulation strokes have significant overlap.[289]

96. Answer c

Fabry disease is an x-linked lysosomal storage disorder caused by mutations to the GLA gene resulting in abnormal activity of the α-galactosidase A enzyme. This leads to accumulation of glycolipids in a range of organs throughout the body.[290]

97. Answer a

Fibrates were developed following the discovery that French farmers exposed to an insecticide had low cholesterol levels. They were the main anti-lipid medications prior to the introduction of statin medications. They act predominantly on plasma triglyceride concentration with a smaller decrease in LDL-C and increase in HDL-C.[291]

98. Answer e

Erysipelothrix rhusiopathiae is a bacterial zoonosis found as a commensal or pathogen in a wide variety of animal species. The main reservoir is domestic pigs, but other animals may also act as a source. The most common clinical manifestation is erysipeloid, a localised cellulitis which usually affects the hands. It may rarely cause endocarditis or septicaemia.[292]

99. Answer e

Chikungunya is an arboviral infection that was initially reported in the 1950s in Tanzania. The name Chikungunya derived from a local term meaning 'that which bends up'. The virus has caused explosive outbreaks in Africa, Asia and the Americas. The clinical presentation is similar to Dengue fever with some important differences. Most of those infected with Chikungunya virus are symptomatic. Fever is of onset within two cays of infection. There may be a maculopapular rash. Severe joint pains are a feature of the infection which can last for months to years after infection has resolved. CNS involvement may occur. Fatality rates vary but are estimated at 1:1000 and the elderly are highest risk. Retro-orbital headache which is a common feature of Dengue fever is conspicuously absent in Chikungunya.[295]

100. Answer b

Idiosyncratic drug-induced liver injury occurs when there are alterations in liver biochemical tests resulting from appropriate use of a drug within recommended dosages. It can vary from mild asymptomatic and self-limiting rise in liver biochemical tests to life-threatening acute liver failure. It can vary from hepatitis to cholestasis, to autoimmune induced liver injury. Several drugs are implicated. Anti-microbials are the most common worldwide although the specific drugs may vary between different countries, with amoxicillin and flucloxacillin common causes in Europe and anti-tuberculous drugs the most common in India.

Mortality rates have been reported from 2% to 14.3% depending on the pattern of liver injury.

Rechallenge can be tried with antituberculous drugs, particularly where combination drugs have been used initially. It may be unclear which drug caused the reaction and practical alternative drugs may not be available for

Treatment. Rechallenge with monitoring may be attempted with specialist supervision.

As no diagnostic markers exist, it is primarily a diagnosis of exclusion.[294]

Paper 4

1. Legionella pneumophila:
    a. Is aerobic
    b. Is gram-positive
    c. Was discovered in the 19th century
    d. Is the only cause of legionellosis
    e. Most people exposed to L pneumophila will develop legionellosis

2. 'Bull's eye' retinopathy is an adverse effect of treatment with:
    a. Methotrexate
    b. Hydroxychloroquine
    c. Ethambutol
    d. Corticosteroids
    e. Amitryptiline

3. Prolactinomas:
    a. Are the most common pituitary adenoma
    b. Size does not usually correlate with level of hyperprolactinaemia
    c. Are always less then 1cm in size
    d. Occur with equal frequency in men and women
    e. First-line treatment is with surgery

4. Hydroxyurea exerts its effects in sickle cell disease by modifying levels of:
    a. HbS
    b. HbA
    c. HbF
    d. HbC
    e. HbD

5. Which of the following interventions are <u>not</u> shown to reduce frequency of exacerbations in chronic obstructive pulmonary disease:

    a.   Influenza vaccination
    b.   Pneumococcal vaccination
    c.   Macrolide antibiotics
    d.   Long term oral steroids
    e.   Inhaled long acting beta-agonists

6. The leading infectious cause of death worldwide is:

    a.   HIV
    b.   Malaria
    c.   Tuberculosis
    d.   Influenza
    e.   Coronavirus

7. Natriuretic peptides:

    a.   Are not useful in heart failure with preserved ejection fraction
    b.   Are not useful in chronic heart failure
    c.   Are not useful to exclude acute heart failure as a cause for shortness of breath
    d.   Raised levels are sufficient to diagnose heart failure and no further testing is needed
    e.   Levels may be more difficult to interpret in the elderly

8. Myasthenia gravis (MG):

    a.   Autoantibodies against muscle specific kinase (MuSK) are the most commonly found in MG
    b.   May require ventilatory support
    c.   Symptoms may improve when taking beta-blockers
    d.   Thymectomy has not been shown to be superior to steroid treatment alone
    e.   Tendon reflexes are reduced

9. Primary syphilis typically presents with a chancre:

    a.   That is painful

    b.   That typically presents at the site of contact with the sexual partner's infectious lesion

    c.   That only presents in the genital area

    d.   That will only heal if treated

    e.   That will heal with scarring

10. Which is the most likely combination of metabolic disturbance seen in primary adrenal insufficiency (Addison's disease):

    a.   Hyponatraemia, hyperkalaemia and hypoglycaemia

    b.   Hypernatraemia, hypokalaemia and hypoglycaemia

    c.   Hyponatraemia, hypokalaemia and hyperglycaemia

    d.   Hypernatraemia, hypokalaemia and hyperglycaemia

    e.   Hypernatremia, hyperkalaemia and hyperglycaemia

11. Lung cancer:

    a.   Risk returns to that of the general population in ex-smokers who stopped smoking 10 or more years previously

    b.   Half of all lung cancers occur in those over 70 years of age

    c.   Risk increases with duration of smoking but not number of cigarettes smoked daily

    d.   Family history of lung cancer does not increase an individual's risk

    e.   A history of previous lung cancer does not increase an individual's risk

12. Influenza:

    a.   Is a zoonosis

    b.   Influenza A occurs exclusively in humans

    c.   Peaks in the southern hemisphere between December and April

    d.   Pandemics are more likely to be caused by influenza B than by influenza A

    e.   Influenza A will not cause acute respiratory distress syndrome

13. The following is the appropriate sequence of benign liver lesions, in order from most common to least common:

    a.   Hepatic haemangioma - hepatic adenoma – focal nodular hyperplasia

    b.   Hepatic haemangioma – focal nodular hyperplasia – hepatic adenoma

    c.   Hepatic adenoma – hepatic haemangioma – focal nodular hyperplasia

    d.   Focal nodular hyperplasia – hepatic adenoma – hepatic haemangioma

    e.   Focal nodular hyperplasia – hepatic haemangioma – hepatic adenoma

14. Corticosteroids:

    a.   Are hormones with 15 carbon atoms

    b.   Have exclusively either glucocorticoid or mineralocorticoid properties

    c.   The main glucocorticoid produced by the adrenal cortex is aldosterone

    d.   The anti-inflammatory potency of corticosteroids is closely related to its potency in carbohydrate metabolism

    e.   Dexamethasone has strong mineralocorticoid effects

15. Which of the following is the most useful feature in the diagnosis of Parkinson's disease:

    a.   Rigidity

    b.   Bradykinesia

    c.   Normal MRI scan of brain

    d.   Response to dopamine agonist

    e.   Absence of dementia

16. The most common endogenous cause of Cushing's syndrome is:

    a.   Congenital adrenal hyperplasia

    b.   Pituitary corticotroph adenoma

    c.   Ectopic corticotroph adenoma

    d.   Adrenal adenoma

    e.   Adrenal carcinoma

17. Pityriasis rosea:

a.   Is associated with human herpesvirus 7 (HHV7)
b.   Can be excluded if the lesions are itchy
c.   Oral lesions do not occur
d.   Should be treated with oral acyclovir
e.   Will not be associated with systemic symptoms

18. Which of the following is the most likely cause of primary hyperparathyroidism:

a.   Malabsorption
b.   Renal impairment
c.   Parathyroid adenoma
d.   Lithium treatment
e.   Vitamin D deficiency

19. Cystic fibrosis:

a.   Staphylococcus aureus is the most commonly isolated respiratory pathogen
b.   Pseudomonas aeruginosa colonisation is not a useful prognostic indicator
c.   Long term macrolide treatment has not been shown to be beneficial
d.   Inhaled antibiotics may reduce exacerbation rates
e.   Long term flucloxacillin use will not reduce staphylococcus aureus infection rates

20. Flecainide:

a.   Does not require echocardiogram prior to administration
b.   Can be given as an 'as needed' medication in paroxysmal atrial fibrillation
c.   Should not be given concomitantly with betablockers
d.   Is less effective than betablockers at converting acute atrial fibrillation to sinus rhythm
e.   Is safe to use in heart failure

21. Hodgkin's lymphoma:
    a. Most commonly presents in the 50-60 year age group
    b. Is best diagnosed by fine needle aspirate of the suspicious lesion
    c. Is excluded by a normal full blood count
    d. The presence of B symptoms is a good prognostic sign
    e. A raised ESR is a poor prognostic sign

22. Which of the following investigations would be most useful when you feel that a diagnosis of Crohn's disease is likely:
    a. CRP
    b. Full blood count
    c. Faecal calprotectin
    d. Ileocolonoscopy
    e. Abdominal ultrasound

23. The most frequent cardiovascular abnormality found in subclinical hypothyroidism is:
    a. Systolic dysfunction
    b. Diastolic dysfunction
    c. Hypertension
    d. Atrial fibrillation
    e. 1st degree heart block

24. Advantages of direct oral anticoagulants over vitamin K antagonists for the treatment of venous thromboembolic disease does not include:
    a. No need for PT/INR monitoring
    b. Longer half-life
    c. Fixed dosage
    d. Reduced risk of major bleeding events
    e. Rapid onset of action

25. Ulcerative colitis:
    a. Most patients have progressive disease
    b. Sulfasalazine is less effective than other 5-ASA preparations
    c. 50% will require surgical intervention at 10 years after diagnosis
    d. Associated primary sclerosing cholangitis indicates milder disease
    e. Older age at onset (>60 years of age) is poor prognostic signs

26. In an adult with new onset hyperglycaemia diagnostic of diabetes mellitus, differentiating between type 1 and type 2 diabetes can be difficult. Where doubt exists, the investigation of choice is:
    a. C peptide
    b. Hb A1c
    c. Glucose tolerance test
    d. Autoantibodies to pancreatic β cells or insulin
    e. Random plasma glucose

27. Infective endocarditis:
    a. Shortness of breath is the most common presenting symptom
    b. Vegetations are always on the ventricular surface of the valve
    c. Serology is usually required for endocarditis in Q fever
    d. New valvular regurgitation in a febrile patient is sufficient for diagnosis
    e. Vegetations will not exceed 1cm in size

28. Idiopathic pulmonary fibrosis:
    a. Is more common in women
    b. Tends to occur in a younger population than other interstitial lung diseases
    c. Is reversible
    d. Progresses to respiratory failure and death within a medial interval of 3 years from diagnosis
    e. Pulmonary function testing typically shows an obstructive pattern

29. Which of the following is most likely to be caused by a transient ischaemic attack:

    a.   Aphasia

    b.   Unilateral facial sensory deficit

    c.   Transient loss of consciousness

    d.   Headache

    e.   Amnesia

30. Positive predictive value of a test refers to:

    a.   The proportion of people with a condition who have a positive test result

    b.   The proportion of people without a condition who have a negative test result

    c.   The proportion of people with a condition with a given test result (either positive or negative) divided by the proportion of people without the condition with that result

    d.   Post-test probability that a person with a positive test result has the condition

    e.   Post-test probability that a person with a negative test result does not have the condition

31. Human respiratory droplets:

    a.   Will not be exhaled during normal speaking

    b.   Can range in size up to 10μm

    c.   Will generally evaporate prior to contact with surfaces

    d.   Droplet size will not affect the severity of an infection transmitted by the droplet

    e.   Aerosol particles (<5μm) may take several hours to settle on a surface

32. The most common autoimmune condition associated with type 1 diabetes is:

    a.   Coeliac disease

    b.   Autoimmune thyroiditis

    c.   Addison's disease

    d.   Rheumatoid arthritis

    e.   Pernicious anaemia

33. Hepatitis C virus is known to have:
    a.   3 genotypes
    b.   4 genotypes
    c.   5 genotypes
    d.   6 genotypes
    e.   7 genotypes

34. Anti-citrullinated protein antibodies (ACPAs):
    a.   Are highly sensitive but not specific for rheumatoid arthritis
    b.   Are IgM isotype only
    c.   Their presence increases the risk of bony erosions in rheumatoid arthritis
    d.   Their detection is sufficient to diagnose rheumatoid arthritis
    e.   Their detection is necessary to diagnose rheumatoid arthritis

35. The most common type of recurring infections occurring in common variable immunodeficiency is:
    a.   Skin infections
    b.   Urinary tract infection
    c.   Gastrointestinal infections
    d.   Respiratory tract infections
    e.   Sepsis

36. Down syndrome:
    a.   Risk of Moyamoya disease is increased
    b.   Thyroid abnormalities will occur in 90% by the age of 45
    c.   Most will have symptoms of Alzheimer's disease by age 40
    d.   Cholinesterase inhibitors have been shown to be effective in dementia in those with Down syndrome
    e.   The most common cause of death is heart failure

37. Transfusion-related acute lung injury (TRALI):
    a.   There may be signs of circulatory overload
    b.   There may be a temporal association with a risk factor for acute respiratory distress syndrome
    c.   Is more likely to occur when the donor is a previously pregnant female
    d.   Occurs only with whole blood transfusion
    e.   Pooling blood products from multiple donors may increase risk

38. The E in CREST syndrome stands for:
    a.   Endocarditis
    b.   Oesophageal dysmotility
    c.   Enophthalmos
    d.   Exophthalmos
    e.   Eye involvement

39. Looser zones are cortical stress fractures perpendicular to the long axis of the bone and are classic radiographic findings of:
    a.   Osteoporosis
    b.   Osteomalacia
    c.   Achondroplasia
    d.   Paget's disease
    e.   Primary hyperparathyroidism

40. Undifferentiated connective tissue disease:
    a.   Occurs when a patient meets the definition for two or more defined autoimmune conditions
    b.   All cases will ultimately be defined as having a single connective tissue disease
    c.   Major organ involvement is usual
    d.   Risk of progression to a defined connective tissue disease is within the first two years
    e.   Non-steroidal anti-inflammatory medications are contraindicated

41. Thrombophilia:

a.   Inherited thrombophilias do not increase venous thromboembolic disease (VTE)

b.   Factor V Leiden heterozygotes do not have increased risk of venous thromboembolic disease

c.   Acquired thrombophilias do not increase risk of venous thromboembolic disease

d.   Recurring venous thromboembolic disease is likely in all those with an inherited thrombophilia

e.   Thrombophilia testing should be considered in younger patients with VTE which are unprovoked who have a strong family history of VTE.

42. The most common porphyria is:

a.   Hereditary coproporphyria

b.   X linked protoporphyria

c.   Porphyria cutanea tarda

d.   Acute intermittent porphyria

e.   Variegate porphyria

43. Hyperthyroidism:

a.   Ophthalmopathy is the least common extrathyroidal manifestation of Graves' disease

b.   Thyroid dermopathy predominantly affects the trunk

c.   Almost all patients with thyroid dermopathy have co-existing ophthalmopathy

d.   Older patients tend to have more pronounced symptoms than younger patients

e.   Those over 60 years of age with hyperthyroidism have 10 times the risk of atrial fibrillation than those with a healthy thyroid

44. Focal motor seizures occur due to an epileptogenic lesion on:

a.   The ipsilateral frontal lobe

b.   The contralateral frontal lobe

c.   The ipsilateral parietal lobe

d.   The contralateral parietal lobe

e.   The contralateral occipital lobe

45. Primary aldosteronism:

a. Renin and angiotensin II levels are high in primary aldosteronism
b. Does not increase the risk of death in blood-pressure matched controls
c. Renal potassium and water reabsorption are increased
d. Most patients will have hypokalaemia
e. Is the most common cause of secondary hypertension

46. Diminished biceps reflex is a sign of nerve root compression at:

a. C3
b. C4
c. C5
d. C6
e. C7

47. The most common positive antibody found in Sjogren's syndrome is:

a. Rheumatoid factor
b. Anti-Ro antibodies
c. Anti-La antibodies
d. Anti U1RNP antibodies
e. Anti-mitochondrial antibodies

48. Chronic lymphocytic leukaemia:

a. All patients require treatment
b. Treatment is not indicated
c. Treatment should be initiated only with a rising lymphocyte count
d. Treatment should be initiated in those with symptomatic or progressive disease
e. Treatment is indicated only in those with recurring infection

49. Pulmonary hypertension:
a. The gold standard modality for diagnosis is transoesophageal echocardiogram
b. Is defined as a pulmonary capillary wedge pressure of >25mmHg
c. May be a heritable disease
d. Will not present with chest pain
e. Treatment is identical irrespective of the cause

50. The most frequent neurological symptom in Wilson's disease is:
a. Tremor
b. Dysarthria
c. Dystonia
d. Chorea
e. Ataxia

51. Serum sodium measurements:
a. Will not be affected by abnormal serum protein levels
b. Pseudohypernatraem a may occur in those with severe hyperlipidaem a
c. Will not be affected by hyperglycaemia
d. Direct measurement of sodium levels with a direct potentiometer such as one of the most modern blood gas analysers) can reliably measure true serum sodium concentration
e. Endocrine causes of hyponatraemia are rare

52. COVID-19:
a. May cause chilblain-like lesions on the hands and feet
b. COVID-19 pneumonia can be excluded with chest x ray
c. Commonly causes lymphocytosis
d. Chest x-ray changes typically affect the upper lobes
e. Causes anosmia in 90% of those affected

53. The initial steroid-sparing agent in the treatment of polymyalgia rheumatica should be:
    a. Hydroxychloroquine
    b. Azathioprine
    c. Methotrexate
    d. Etanercept
    e. Infliximab

54. Postural orthostatic tachycardia syndrome (POTS):
    a. Requires a sustained rise in heart rate of at least 10bpm on assuming the upright posture
    b. Requires a sustained rise in heart rate of at least 20bpm on assuming the upright posture
    c. Requires a sustained rise in heart rate of at least 30bpm on assuming the upright posture
    d. Requires a sustained rise in heart rate of at least 40bpm on assuming the upright posture
    e. Requires a sustained rise in heart rate of at least 50bpm on assuming the upright posture

55. The first-line medical treatment in trigeminal neuralgia is:
    a. Carbamazepine
    b. Pregabalin
    c. Gabapentin
    d. Amitryptiline
    e. Duloxetine

56. Which of the following are not radiological features suggestive of malignancy on ultrasound of lymph nodes:
    a. Microcalcifications
    b. Hyperechogenicity
    c. Peripheral vascularity
    d. Oval shape
    e. Cystic aspect

57. Primary biliary cirrhosis:

    a.   Anti-mitochondrial antibodies are always positive

    b.   Aminotransferase levels are usually normal

    c.   IgG is the most commonly elevated immunoglobulin

    d.   The Mayo risk score is the most reliable prognostic system

    e.   No treatment improves patient survival

58. The QT interval:

    a.   Is the same in all leads of a 12 lead ECG

    b.   A U wave, if present, should be included in the QT interval measurement

    c.   Correction for heart rate is not necessary

    d.   Should be calculated from a single QRS complex

    e.   When studied it was found that the majority of physicians cannot recognise a long QT when they see one

59. Clostridioides difficile infection (CDI):

    a.   Does not occur in those under the age of 65

    b.   Risk is higher during antibiotic treatment but returns to normal one week after completon of an antibiotic course

    c.   Community acquired CDI does not occur

    d.   Clostridioides difficile spores survive in the environment for several months

    e.   Gastric acid kills clostridioides difficile

60. Upper extremity deep vein thrombosis (UEDVT):

    a.   Wells score has been validated in UEDVT

    b.   D Dimer is useful to excluding the diagnosis in those with a low clinical probability of UEDVT

    c.   Ultrasonography is not useful in diagnosis

    d.   Lifelong anticoagulation is required in all patients with UEDVT

    e.   Direct oral anticoagulants are contraindicated in UEDVT

61. Gastric antral vascular ectasia (GAVE):
    a.   Is an inherited disorder
    b.   Is more common in males
    c.   Most of those affected will not require blood transfusion
    d.   Is diagnosed by the endoscopic appearance of the gastric wall
    e.   Long term steroids normalise the endoscopic appearance of the stomach

62. The most common form of dementia presenting in those over 65 years of age is:
    a.   Alzheimer's disease
    b.   Lewy body dementia
    c.   Vascular dementia
    d.   Frontotemporal dementia
    e.   Progressive supranuclear palsy

63. Which of the following is not a risk factor for bleeding on anticoagulation:
    a.   Uncontrolled hypertension with systolic blood pressure >160mmHg
    b.   History of prior major bleeding
    c.   Associated use of non-steroidal anti-inflammatory medications
    d.   Alcohol use of 8 drinks or more per week
    e.   Risk of falling

64. Herpes zoster (shingles):
    a.   Rash extent is not a risk factor for post herpetic neuralgia
    b.   There is an increased risk of vascular events in the months following shingles
    c.   Where laboratory diagnosis may be required, viral culture is the gold standard
    d.   Corticosteroid treatment reduces the incidence of post herpetic neuralgia
    e.   Famciclovir has been shown to be more effective than acyclovir and valaciclovir

65. Bullous pemphigoid:

a. Is less common than pemphigus
b. Is more likely to occur in those under than over the age of 70 years of age
c. Requires the presence of blisters for diagnosis
d. Lesions are not usually itchy
e. There is an increased risk of venous thromboembolic disease

66. The definition of acute kidney injury includes an increase in serum creatinine of at least:

a. 1.5 times baseline in seven days
b. 2 times baseline in seven days
c. 2.5 times baseline in seven days
d. 3 times baseline in seven days
e. 3.5 times baseline in seven days

67. Stroke:

a. Antiplatelet therapy should be avoided in the first 24 hours after TIA or minor stroke
b. Dual antiplatelet therapy reduces risk of stroke compared to single antiplatelet therapy after minor stroke or TIA
c. 50% of people will have a stroke within 90 days after a minor stroke or TIA
d. Antiplatelet therapy is permanently contraindicated after a haemorrhagic stroke
e. $ABCD_2$ score should be used after all those with TIA to assess risk of stroke

68. Long term urate lowering treatment in gout:

a. Can be started during an acute attack
b. Should be avoided in nephrolithiasis
c. Should be avoided in renal impairment
d. Should be avoided in transplant recipients
e. Should be stopped during an acute attack

69. Bell's palsy:
   a. All those affected should be tested for Lyme disease
   b. Corticosteroids have no role in treatment
   c. Surgery has no role in treatment
   d. 1% will have permanent facial weakness
   e. Should be treated with antivirals

70. Corticosteroids for acute exacerbations of COPD should be continued for:
   a. 2-4 days
   b. 5-7 days
   c. 7-10 days
   d. 10-14 days
   e. >14 days

71. Stage 5 chronic kidney disease, also known as end-stage renal disease is classified as disease with glomerular filtration rate of:
   a. $<90ml/min/1.73m^2$
   b. $<60ml/min/1.73m^2$
   c. $<45ml/min/1.73m^2$
   d. $<15ml/min/1.73m^2$
   e. $<5ml/min/1.73m^2$

72. The percentage of people with DVT subsequently diagnosed with cancer is:
   a. 10%
   b. 30%
   c. 50%
   d. 70%
   e. 90%

73. The investigation required for diagnosis of autoimmune hepatitis is:
    a. ANA antibodies
    b. Anti smooth muscle antibodies
    c. Serum immunoglobulins
    d. Liver ultrasound
    e. Liver biopsy

74. Familial hypercholesterolaemia in its most common form:
    a. Is polygenic
    b. Is autosomal recessive
    c. Causes premature cardiovascular disease due to high triglyceride levels
    d. There is no gene dosage effect
    e. Is caused by the LDL receptor having decreased capacity to clear LDL from the per pheral circulation

75. Versive seizures consist of:
    a. Collapse with loss of consciousness and repeated short contractions of various muscle groups
    b. Repeated short contractions of various muscle groups lasting less than 1 to 2 seconds
    c. Sustained contractions of various muscle groups lasting more than 5 to 10 seconds resulting in posturing of the limbs and whole body
    d. Sustained, forceful, involuntary turning of the head and eyes to one side due to tonic contraction of the head and eye muscles
    e. Repetitive contractions in one hand progressing up one arm and to the ipsilateral foot and leg

76. Velcro rales are heard in:
    a. Heart failure
    b. Pneumonia
    c. Pulmonary fibrosis
    d. Bronchiectasis
    e. Lung malignancy

77. Darier disease:
    a. Is autosomal dominant
    b. Has low penetrance in those affected
    c. Is more frequent in women
    d. Acantholysis does not occur
    e. Is caused by a mutation in the ATP2C1 gene

78. Which of the following is not a clinical feature of complex regional pain syndrome (CRPS):
    a. Changes in skin temperature and colour,
    b. Oedema
    c. Hyperalgesia
    d. Allodynia
    e. Pain occurring in a dermatomal distribution

79. Benign paroxysmal positional vertigo:
    a. May occur secondary to Meniere's disease
    b. The horizontal semicircular canal variant is the most common
    c. If symptoms occur when turning the head to the left when lying flat, it implies the right inner ear is involved
    d. Vertigo usually lasts more than one minute
    e. Hanging the head over the back if the bed on lying flat is necessary when performing Dix-Hallpike manoeuvre

80. Which of the following autoantibodies is associated with mixed connective tissue disorder:
    a. Anti-synthetase Ab
    b. Anti CCP Ab
    c. Anti-U1RNP
    d. Anti PM-Scl Ab
    e. Anti-SSA/B

81. The most common subtype of Guillain Barre syndrome is:
    a. Acute motor axonal neuropathy
    b. Acute motor sensory axonal neuropathy
    c. Acute inflammatory demyelinating polyradiculopathy
    d. Miller Fischer syndrome
    e. Acute autonomic neuropathy

82. The most common cause of ascending cholangitis is:
    a. Pancreatic cancer
    b. Liver cirrhosis
    c. Biliary stent obstruction
    d. Post endoscopic retrograde cholangiopancreatography (ERCP)
    e. Gallstones

83. Lowering LDL-C levels by 2mmol/L has been associated with a reduction in cardiovascular events by:
    a. 15%
    b. 25%
    c. 35%
    d. 45%
    e. 55%

84. Autosomal dominant polycystic kidney disease (ADPKD):
    a. Intracranial aneurysms are detected in 50% of patients
    b. Intracranial aneurysms are more common than the general population but the median age of rupture is the same as the general population
    c. Presymptomatic screening for intracranial aneurysms is recommended for all patients with ADPKD
    d. Family history of intracranial aneurysm further increases the risk of intracranial aneurysm in those with ADPKD
    e. Anterior location of the intracranial aneurysm increases risk of rupture

85. Which of the following is a useful treatment for von Willebrand's disease:
    a.   Desmopressin
    b.   Spironolactone
    c.   Bisoprolol
    d.   Hydroxocobalamin
    e.   Warfarin

86. Current recommendations for the diagnosis of type 1 or type 2 diabetes as per World Health Organisation and American Diabetes Association criteria include a Hb A1c greater than or equal to:
    a.   42mmol/mol
    b.   46mmol/mol
    c.   48mmol/mol
    d.   50mmol/mol
    e.   53mmol/mol

87. Chronic kidney disease:
    a.   Albumin-to-creatinine ratio of >30 ml/min/1.73m^{2}for three months is to demonstrate kidney damage in chronic kidney disease
    b.   Most cases will spontaneously improve
    c.   A single episode of acute kidney injury does not increase risk of chronic kidney disease
    d.   The principal cause of morbidity and mortality in those with chronic kidney disease is end stage renal disease
    e.   Dual renin-angiotensin-aldosterone system blockade with ACE inhibitors and angiotensin receptor blockers has been shown to reduce cardiovascular mortality in those with chronic kidney disease

88. Skin prick testing:
    a.   A positive reaction is a wheal of mean diameter >10mm
    b.   A positive reaction always indicates allergy
    c.   Results are always consistent with RAST blood testing
    d.   It is useful in assessing sensitization to any IgE-mediated allergic disease
    e.   There is a 5% risk of anaphylaxis arising from a skin prick test

89. In COVID-19, serum IgG antibody secretion occurs how soon after onset of symptoms:
    a.   Days 1-4
    b.   Days 5-7
    c.   Days 7-10
    d.   Days 11-14
    e.   Days 14-21

90. The most reliable way of diagnosing herpes simplex encephalitis is:
    a.   MRI brain
    b.   Serology
    c.   Cerebrospinal protein and white blood cell analysis
    d.   CSF PCR
    e.   CSF RT-PCR

91. Interferon-γ-release assays:
    a.   Detect IgG antibodies to tuberculosis
    b.   Can differentiate between those with latent tuberculosis and previous BCG vaccination
    c.   Can differentiate between those with latent tuberculosis and active tuberculosis
    d.   Can differentiate between those with latent tuberculosis and all other non-tuberculous mycobacterial infections
    e.   Can predict who will progress from latent to active tuberculosis

92. West Nile virus:
    a.   Rash is not a feature of West Nile fever
    b.   Case fatality rate is 50% for neuroinvasive disease
    c.   Return to baseline function is usual 6 months after neuroinvasive disease
    d.   Recent yellow fever vaccination may produce a false positive serum antibody test
    e.   IgM antibody to West Nile virus is not usually isolated from cerebrospinal flu d in neuroinvasive disease

93. Hepatitis E virus:
   a. Does not occur in industrialised countries
   b. Does not cause liver failure
   c. Sheep are the main zoonotic reservoir
   d. Presents a higher risk for pregnant women than for the non-pregnant population
   e. No vaccine exists

94. The definition of acute kidney injury includes an increase in serum creatinine of at least:
   a. 0.1 mg/dL (8.84 µmol/L) in 48 hours
   b. 0.2 mg/dL (17.68 µmol/L) in 48 hours
   c. 0.3 mg/dL (26.53 µmol/L) in 48 hours
   d. 0.4 mg/dL (35.37 µmol/L) in 48 hours
   e. 0.5 mg/dL (44.21 µmol//L) in 48 hours

95. Gout:
   a. Always requires joint fluid analysis for diagnosis
   b. Raised white bloods cells and inflammatory markers are uncommon in acute gout
   c. Serum uric acid will be at its highest during an acute gout attack
   d. Acute flares are caused by calcium pyrophosphate crystal deposition
   e. Statins should be stopped during colchicine treatment

96. Posterior circulation stroke:
   a. Does not cause limb paresis
   b. Cannot be treated with tissue plasminogen activator
   c. The best radiological test for detection is CT scan
   d. Risk of stroke after posterior circulation TIA is at least as high as after anterior circulation TIA
   e. The FAST score has greater sensitivity for pre-hospital assessment in posterior circulation stroke than for anterior circulation stroke

97. Fabry disease:

 a. Is autosomal dominant
 b. Cannot be tested for on dried blood spots
 c. Demonstration of normal levels of the affected enzyme α-galactosidase A are sufficient to exclude the diagnosis in males and females
 d. Clinical features may present in childhood or adulthood
 e. The deficient enzyme cannot be replaced

98. Fibrates:

 a. May reduce cardiovascular events
 b. May reduce all-cause mortality
 c. May reduce cardiovascular mortality
 d. Are shown to reduce cardiovascular endpoints in primary prevention when combined with a statin
 e. Should be used as monotherapy if a statin is not well tolerated

99. Latent autoimmune diabetes of adulthood (LADA):

 a. Will not present with ketoacidosis
 b. Will not require insulin treatment
 c. Is best managed with oral hypoglycaemics
 d. Peak incidence is at age 25
 e. Requires the presence of at least one circulating autoantibody associated with type 1 diabetes mellitus

100. Which of the following is not a typical clinical feature of Chikungunya:

 a. Fever
 b. Maculopapular rash
 c. Severe joint pains
 d. Retro-orbital headache
 e. Vomiting

1. Answer a

Legionella pneumophila is an aerobic gram-negative bacterium, discovered following an outbreak of disease at an American Legion Conference in Philadelphia in 1976. It is found in bodies of water and is a common cause of atypical pneumonia. It causes 90% of legionellosis (or Legionnaire's disease). Other Legionella serotypes cause the remainder. Less than 5% of those exposed in the community will develop legionellosis.[39]

2. Answer b

Hydroxychloroquine is used in rheumatological conditions such as systemic lupus erythematosus and rheumatoid arthritis. Long-term use of both chloroquine and its analogue hydroxychloroquine can cause damage to the retinal pigment epithelium, with an area of depigmentation and central foveal sparing on fundoscopy resulting in the 'bull's eye' appearance. Severe retinopathy causes visual impairment and is irreversible, and may progress even after the medication is stopped. Risk increases with prolonged treatment at higher dosages. Regular ophthalmological screening is recommended for any individual who is on this medication long term.[47]

Ethambutol is an anti-tuberculosis medication known to cause visual impairment due to optic neuritis.

Corticosteroids are associated with increased risk of cataract.

Amitryptiline and other tricyclic antidepressants are linked with an increased risk of acute glaucoma (although rare).

3. Answer a

Prolactinomas are the most common pituitary adenoma. They may be microprolactinomas (less than 1cm) or macroprolactinomas (1cm or larger). The level of hyperprolactinaemia is usually related to the size of prolactinoma in non-cystic lesions although there may be exceptions. Prolactinomas are more common in women. First-line treatment is with dopamine agonists although surgery may be needed in some cases.[50]

4. Answer c

Hydroxyurea is an anti-neoplastic agent used to treat myeloproliferative disorders and leukaemia. It is also used in sickle cell disease to increase HbF levels. HbF (fetal haemoglobin) levels are low in most individuals, but tend to be higher in those with sickle cell disease. It is excluded from the polymerisation of HbS which occurs in sickle cell disease and high HbF levels are associated with less severe disease.[48,51,52]

5. Answer d

Influenza vaccination has been shown to reduce exacerbations of COPD as well as hospitalisation due to lower respiratory tract infection. Pneumococcal vaccination has also been shown to reduce exacerbations with moderate quality evidence. Inhaled long acting beta-agonists and long acting muscarinic antagonists are also shown to reduce exacerbations as well as improving lung function and symptom scores. Macrolide antibiotics have been shown to reduce exacerbations by up to 27%. Long term oral steroids have not been shown to have any benefit in reducing exacerbation rate.[53]

6. Answer c

Tuberculosis is the leading infectious cause of death worldwide.[54]

7. Answer e

Natriuretic peptides are raised in heart failure due to ventricular overload. They consist of brain natriuretic peptide (BNP) and N-terminal pro-BNP (NT-proBNP). Their use is most established at present in acute heart failure in the hospital setting. They have a high negative predictive value, so can be useful for excluding acute heart failure as a cause of shortness of breath. They can be useful for both heart failure with reduced and preserved ejection fraction. Their sensitivity is modest and follow up testing such as echocardiogram is needed. Levels are raised in chronic heart failure also but their use is less well established in this setting. Levels can be more difficult to interpret in certain populations, such as the elderly where levels can be raised for non-cardiac reasons, and in obesity where levels may be reduced.[56,57,58]

8. Answer b

Myasthenia gravis is an autoimmune condition characterised by muscle fatiguability. Pathological autoantibodies have been identified such as against acetylcholine receptors (AChRs – 85% of cases), muscle-specific kinase (MuSK – 10% of cases) and lipoprotein related protein 4 (LPR4). Symptoms can worsen with certain triggers such as pregnancy, hypokalaemia, infection and medications including beta-blockers. Tendon reflexes are normal. Treatments include symptomatic treatment with pyridostigmine, immunosuppression with steroids or steroid-sparing agents such as azathioprine. Thymectomy has been shown to be superior to steroids alone. Ventilatory support may be needed with myasthenic crisis during a relapse.[23,64,65]

9. Answer b

Primary syphilis typically presents with a painless chancre in the genital area at the point of contact with the sexual partner's lesion. It may present in extragenital areas such as the mouth or anus. It will heal without scarring even without treatment with penicillin.[69,70]

10. Answer a

Primary adrenal insufficiency is most likely to lead to hyponatraemia, hyperkalaemia and hypoglycaemia, with hypoglycaemia more common in children than adults.[73,74,75]

11. Answer b

Smoking is the predominant risk factor for lung cancer and increased risk persists in ex-smokers. Risk also increases with age and half of all lung cancers occur in those over 70 years of age. The increased risk of lung cancer in smokers is dose-dependent and increases with both duration of smoking and number of cigarettes smoked per day. First-degree relatives of an individual with lung cancer have a two-fold increased risk. Multiple family members with lung cancer at a younger age increases an individual's risk. A history of previous lung cancer also increases risk of second metachronous cancer.[76]

12. Answer a

Influenza B occurs almost exclusively in humans while influenza A occurs in both humans and a large array of animal hosts with the potential for cross-species infection, and so it is a zoonosis. Influenza infections tend to peak in the winter months which is between June and September in the southern hemisphere. In tropical and subtropical regions seasonal variations are less well defined. Pandemics are more likely to be caused by influenza A due to its numerous animal hosts as well as its tendency towards antigenic shift and antigenic drift. Influenza usually causes a self-limiting respiratory illness but may cause a viral pneumonia progressing to acute respiratory distress syndrome and respiratory failure.[79]

13. Answer b

In descending order, the most common benign liver lesions are hepatic haemangiomas, focal nodular hyperplasia and hepatic adenomas. Hepatic haemangiomas are dilated vascular malformations. Focal nodular hyperplasia are areas of hyperplasia felt to be due to haemodisruption within the liver parenchyma. Hepatic adenomas are areas of benign nodules of proliferating hepatocytes, with a small risk of haemorrhage or malignant transformation.[88]

14. Answer d

Corticosteroids are hormones with 21 carbon atoms. Corticosteroids can be classified as preferentially glucocorticoid (involved in carbohydrate metabolism) or mineralocorticoid (involved in fluid and electrolyte balance), but these properties are not exclusive and many corticosteroids have both properties. The main glucocorticoid produced by the adrenal cortex is cortisol and the main mineralocorticoid produced by the adrenal cortex is aldosterone. The anti-inflammatory potency of corticosteroids is closely related to its potency in carbohydrate metabolism as the glucocorticoid receptors involved act in both functions. Synthetic steroids were originally developed to maximise anti-inflammatory potency, and fluorinated synthetic corticosteroids such as dexamethasone have no mineralocorticoid effects.[93]

15. Answer b

Parkinson's disease is a clinical diagnosis based on the presence of bradykinesia, resting tremor +/- rigidity. Response to dopaminergic medication can be supportive of the diagnosis. Other investigations are generally used to exclude other causes when the diagnosis is in doubt. Neuroimaging such as dopamine transporter single-photon emission computed tomography (DAT-SPECT) or flouro-dopa positron emission tomography (PET) are used to demonstrate dopamine deficit where there is diagnostic uncertainty.[104]

16. Answer b

Cushing's disease refers to hypercortisolism resulting from a corticotroph adenoma, usually in the pituitary. Cushing's syndrome refers to hypercortisolism arising from any cause. Of the endogenous causes corticotroph adenomas are the most common with adrenal sources accounting for the remainder.[198,112]

17. Answer a

Pityriasis rosea is a self-limiting rash thought to be triggered by systemic reactivation of human herpesvirus (HHV) 6 and/or HHV 7. It begins with an erythematous scaly herald patch which may be present for two weeks prior to onset of a more generalised rash consisting of smaller scaly papulosquamous lesions mainly on the trunk. It occurs in adults and children and there is an even gender distribution. 25% are not itchy, 50% mildly itchy and 25% severely itchy. Variable oral lesions may occur in 16% of patients. The rash may be preceded by mild systemic symptoms such as fever and malaise. Oral acyclovir is not routinely used in self-limiting episodes due to a lack of evidence at present.[120]

18. Answer c

Parathyroid adenoma causes 80% of cases of primary hyperparathyroidism. Lithium treatment can cause a clinical picture clinically indistinguishable from primary hyperparathyroidism. Malabsorption, renal impairment and vitamin D deficiency are all causes of secondary hyperparathyroidism.[122]

19. Answer d

Staphylococcus aureus and haemophilus influenza are common respiratory pathogens in early cystic fibrosis but the most commonly isolated respiratory pathogen in cystic fibrosis is pseudomonas aeruginosa. Colonisation with pseudomonas aeruginosa is one the most important predictors of morbidity and mortality in cystic fibrosis. Long term flucloxacillin is used to reduce staphylococcus aureus infection rates in children with cystic fibrosis. Long term treatment with azithromycin has been shown to reduce exacerbation rates and antibiotic use and improve lung function, particularly in those colonised with pseucomonas aeruginosa. Inhaled and nebulised antibiotics such as tobramycin and colomycin to eradicate or reduce pseudomonas aeruginosa colonisation may improve lung function and reduce exacerbation rates.[123]

20. Answer b

Flecainide is a Vaughan-Williams Class IC agent. It has a negative inotropic effect and it is contraindicated in those with reduced ejection fraction or heart failure. Placebo-controlled trials have shown its efficacy in conversion of acute atrial fibrillation to sinus rhythm and also in maintenance of sinus rhythm in those with a history of atrial fibrillation. An echocardiogram should be performed prior to its administration to ensure a structurally normal heart. Beta blockers alone are rarely effective in the acute conversion of atrial fibrillation to sinus rhythm or in prevention of recurrence of atrial fibrillation in patients without heart failure. It can be used as an 'as needed' basis in those with symptomatic recurrences of atrial fibrillation.[124]

21. Answer e

Hodgkin's lymphoma is a malignancy arising from germinal centre and post-germinal centre B cells. It is characterised by the presence of multinucleate giant cells or large mononuclear cells known as Hodgkin and Reed Sternberg (HRS) cells. It can present at any age but is most common in the 20 to 34 year age group which make up one third of new diagnoses. It is best diagnosed by excisional biopsy, as smaller biopsy may miss Hodgkin and Reed Sternberg cells and other histological features. Fine needle aspirate does not establish histological architecture so is not suitable for diagnosis.

Full blood count is only abnormal in late disease. B symptoms include night sweats, fevers and unexplained weight loss of over 10% of body weight. Poor prognostic signs include an elevated ESR, presence of B symptoms, increased number of involved nodal sites and tumour bulk greater than 10cm.[129,130]

22. Answer d

Faecal calprotectin may be useful to exclude inflammatory bowel disease where you feel the diagnosis is unlikely, with sensitivity ranging from 83-100% depending on the cut-off used. Radiology such as CT enterography or MR enterography may also be useful if available. Abdominal ultrasound could also be useful although it is operator dependent and may be limited by body habitus. However in a significantly symptomatic patient where you feel the diagnosis is likely, ileocolonoscopy will provide direct views of the most commonly affected areas of the gastrointestinal tract in Crohn's disease and also allow for a biopsy to be obtained to further aid diagnosis.[131]

23. Answer b

Subclinical hypothyroidism is characterised by raised TSH and normal thyroid hormone levels. Overt hypothyroidism is associated with reduced heart rate, diastolic dysfunction and increased peripheral resistance. The most common cardiovascular abnormality found in subclinical hypothyroidism is diastolic dysfunction due to impaired ventricular filling and relaxation. However the effects of subclinical hypothyroidism on cardiovascular morbidity and mortality are unclear with studies showing conflicting results, and opinions vary as to whether subclinical hypothyroidism should be treated.[134]

24. Answer b

Direct oral anticoagulant (DOAC) medications have been shown to be non-inferior to vitamin K antagonists such as warfarin in the treatment of venous thromboembolic disease. Their advantages include fixed dosage, no need for PT/INR monitoring, reduced risk of major bleeding events, shorter half-life and more rapid onset of action.[136]

25. Answer d

Ulcerative colitis is a chronic inflammatory bowel disease affecting the colon. Most patients have a relapsing remitting disease, and 15% will have severe disease at presentation. Poor prognostic signs include young age at presentation, as well as pancolitis, deep ulceration and failure of endoscopic healing with clinical remission. Presentation over the age of 60 years tends to be associated with a milder course. Associated primary sclerosing cholangitis may be a separate clinical condition, as it tends to be associated with more extensive but milder disease with rectal sparing and ileal involvement. Treatment involves inducing remission, initially with 5 ASA medications followed by steroids if needed. Both can be given topically or systemically, with rectal preparations preferred for disease localised to the rectum. Sulfasalazine is as effective as 5 ASA but is less well tolerated. The need for surgical intervention has been decreasing with 15% requiring surgery at 10 years after diagnosis.[142]

26. Answer d

Differentiating type 1 from type 2 diabetes in adults can be quite difficult as 40% of new cases of type 1 diabetes occur in patients over the age of 30 years. The test of choice is by checking for autoantibodies to pancreatic β cells or insulin. There are several types with anti-glutamic acid decarboxylase autoantibodies (anti-GAD) having the highest diagnostic sensitivity.[273]

27. Answer c

Infective endocarditis (IE) is a multisystem disease arising from infection of the endocardium of the heart. Fever is the most common presenting symptom. Vegetations are usually on the ventricular surface of the aortic or pulmonary valves or atrial surface of the mitral or tricuspid valves. Vegetations may reach several centimetres in size. Coxiella burnetii, the causative organism in Q fever will usually require serology for diagnosis. Diagnosis of endocarditis is made using Duke's criteria, with echocardiography and blood cultures constituting major criteria and clinical features and some risk factors making up minor criteria. Two major criteria, one major and three minor criteria, or five minor criteria are required for diagnosis of definite infective endocarditis. Fever is not one of the criteria.[143,144]

28. Answer d

Idiopathic pulmonary fibrosis occurs more commonly in men than women and is more common over the age of 60 years. Other interstitial lung diseases tend to have a more even gender distribution and are more common in a younger population. The path of idiopathic pulmonary fibrosis is a gradual irreversible worsening of lung function. Pulmonary function testing usually shows a restrictive pattern. Progression to respiratory failure and death occurs within a medial interval of three years after diagnosis.[260]

29. Answer a

Transient ischaemic attack (TIA) involves transient neurological signs or symptoms usually lasting seconds to minutes and usually less than one hour, with no radiological signs of an acute ischaemic infarct on brain radiology. Transient ischaemic attack (TIA) symptoms are likely to be motor, sensory (for example motor or sensory deficit in two limbs or one limb and the face) or visual (monocular blindness or homonymous hemianopia), or involve speech disturbance such as aphasia or dysarthria. Less specific neurological symptoms such as headache, unilateral facial sensory changes, amnesia and transient loss of consciousness are much less likely to be cause by a TIA.[150]

30. Answer d

The positive predictive value of a test refers to the post-test probability that a person with a positive test result has the condition. It can be calculated as:

True positives/ (true positives + false positives)

The proportion of people with a condition who have a positive test result is the sensitivity of a test.

The proportion of people without a condition who have a negative test result is the specificity of a test.

The proportion of people with a condition with a given test result (either positive or negative) divided by the proportion of people without the condition with that result is the likelihood ratio.

The post-test probability that a person with a negative test result does not have the condition is the negative predictive value.[151]

31. Answer e

Human respiratory droplets are exhaled during breathing, speaking, coughing and sneezing. They can range in size from 0.1 to 1000µm. Most respiratory droplets will settle on a surface prior to evaporation. Smaller aerosols (<5µm) are less likely to settle and can be transmitted by air currents for significant distances. A 100µm droplet is predicted to settle to the ground in 4.6 seconds while a 1µm aerosol is predicted to settle in 12.4 hours. Aerosols have also been associated with more severe infection when transmitting influenza virus.[159]

32. Answer b

People with type 1 diabetes have an increased risk of developing other autoimmune conditions. The most common autoimmune disease associated with type 1 diabetes is autoimmune thyroiditis (ie, Hashimoto thyroiditis and Graves' disease) followed by coeliac disease.[161]

33. Answer d

Hepatitis C virus is known to have 6 genotypes. Genotype 3 has a faster progression to cirrhosis and may be less responsive to antiviral treatment. Genotype influences the antiviral treatment regimen used in hepatitis C infection.[162,163]

34. Answer c

Anti-citrullinated protein antibodies (ACPAs) and rheumatoid factor are the main antibodies associated with rheumatoid arthritis, and their presence indicates seropositive rheumatoid arthritis. ACPAs can be IgG, IgA or IgM isotype. They are found in 60-80% of those with rheumatoid arthritis and have a very high specificity of 85-99% for rheumatod arthritis. Their presence is neither sufficient nor necessary for the diagnosis of rheumatoid arthritis, but does have prognostic significance, in particular an increased risk of bony erosions.[164,165]

35. Answer d

Common variable immunodeficiency is characterised by hypogammaglobulinemia and recurrent infections. Respiratory infections are the most common type of recurrent infection with bronchiectasis and interstitial lung disease occurring as a result.[171,174]

36. Answer a

Thyroid abnormalities are common in Down syndrome and occur in 50% by age 45. Most will have histopathological signs of Alzheimer's disease by age 40 but symptoms of cognitive impairment will not develop until they are much older in most. Dementia is more common in those who have seizures. Cholinesterase inhibitors and memantine have not been shown to be effective in dementia in Down syndrome. The most common cause of death in children and adults with Down syndrome is respiratory infection.

Moyamoya disease occurs due to stenosis of the internal carotid arteries and is more common in Down syndrome than the general population. It may present with alternating hemiplegia or a fixed stroke-like deficit.[175]

37. Answer c

Transfusion-related acute lung injury (TRALI) is defined as onset of acute pulmonary oedema within 6 hours of completion of blood product transfusion without circulatory overload or acute respiratory distress syndrome (ARDS) risk factors Where there is a temporal relationship with an ARDS risk factors this is known as possible TRALI. It is thought to be antibody mediated and can occur with transfusion of any blood product. It is more likely to occur when the blood product source is a previously pregnant female due to pregnancy related alloimmunisation. Mitigation of risk is possible through male-only blood product sources, screening donors for antibodies and through pooling blood products from many donors, which dilutes any antibodies present.[176]

38. Answer b

Scleroderma is a connective tissue disease characterised by micro vascular damage and excessive deposition of collagen in the skin and internal organs. It is divided into a localised form (morphoea) which affects the skin only, and a generalised form known as systemic sclerosis. Systemic sclerosis is further subdivided into limited cutaneous systemic scleroderma (lcSSc or CREST syndrome) and diffuse cutaneous systemic scleroderma (dcSSc). These have separate clinical features and are associated with different serological positivity. CREST syndrome is associated with positive anticentromere antibodies and dcSSc is associated with positive antipoisomerase and anti-RNAP III antibodies. CREST syndrome stands for calcinosis, Raynaud's phenomenon , oesophageal involvement, skin sclerosis confined to the fingers and face, and telangiectasia.[266]

39. Answer b

Looser zones are cortical stress fractures perpendicular to the long axis of the bone and are classic radiographic findings of osteomalacia.[177]

40. Answer d

At present five different types of connective tissue disease can be classified: systemic lupus erythematosus, scleroderma, myositis, rheumatoid arthritis and Sjogren's syndrome. Undifferentiated connective tissue disease (UCTD) occurs when a person has features of a connective tissue disease, such as positive anti-nuclear antibody, arthralgia and myalgias and Raynaud's phenomenon, but do not meet the criteria for a specific defined connective tissue disorder. Studies of such groups have shown that approximately 30% of those with UCTD will progress to a defined condition with risk highest in the first two years after diagnosis. In undifferentiated cases major organ involvement is unusual. Treatment can be considered for symptom treatment with NSAIDs for arthralgias, calcium channel blockers for Raynaud's symptoms or hydroxychloroquine for musculoskeletal symptoms.[264]

41. Answer e

Thrombophilias are inherited or acquired blood conditions that increase the propensity for vascular thrombosis. The most common inherited thrombophilias are factor V Leiden and prothrombin gene FII G20210A polymorphism (PGM). Deficiencies in protein C, protein S and antithrombin are less common inherited thrombophilias. The most common acquired thrombophilia is antiphospholipid syndrome.

All thrombophilias, including factor V Leiden and PGM heterozygotes have increased risk of venous thromboembolic events. There is less certainty as to whether all those with thrombophilia are at increased risk of recurring VTE events, and thrombophilia testing is not recommended routinely in VTE as it does not change management. Decisions regarding duration of anticoagulation should be based on the index VTE event, such as whether the event was provoked or unprovoked, bleeding risk and family history. Thrombophilia testing should be considered in those with recurring events at a young age, unusual sites for VTE and a strong family history.[179]

42. Answer c

Porphyrias consist of nine conditions characterised by alterations in enzymes involved in heme biosynthesis. Porphyria cutanea tarda is the most common form, presenting usually as a blistering skin rash in sun exposed areas. It does not have neurological manifestations. Acute intermittent porphyria is the most common acute form of porphyria.[181]

43. Answer c

Ophthalmopathy occurs in 25% of those with Graves' disease. Thyroid acropachy, a clubbing of the fingers and toes, is the least common extrathyroidal manifestation of Graves' disease. Thyroid dermopathy occurs in 1-4% of those with thyroid ophthalmopathy, and almost all those with dermopathy have ophthalmopathy. Thyroid dermopathy manifests as slightly thickened and pigmented skin mainly involving the pretibial area. Younger patients with hyperthyroidism tend to have more pronounced physical symptoms. Those over 60 years of age with hyperthyroidism have three times the risk of atrial fibrillation than those with a healthy thyroid.[188]

44. Answer b

Focal motor seizures occur due to an epileptogenic lesion on the contralateral frontal lobe.[259]

45. Answer e

Primary aldosteronism occurs due to excess aldosterone levels in spite of a sodium and volume avid state where renin and angiotensin II levels are suppressed. Renal sodium and water reabsorption is increased. Hypokalaemia is a feature but present in a minority of individuals. It is the most common cause of secondary hypertension. It is estimated to cause 20% of cases of refractory hypertension. There is an increased risk of mortality even when compared with a blood pressure matched population.[192,193]

46. Answer d

C6 nerve compression causes diminished biceps tendon reflex. Compression at C7 will cause diminished triceps reflex.[198]

47. Answer a

Sjogren's syndrome is characterised by dry mouth and eyes (keratoconjunctivitis sicca) and a variety of extraglandular features. It may be primary or secondary to another chronic inflammatory disease such as SLE or rheumatoid arthritis. Anti-Ro antibodies are found in 60% and anti-La antibodies are found in 40%. Rheumatoid factor is positive in 80% of cases.[265]

48. Answer d

Chronic lymphocytic leukaemia is a malignancy of CD5+ lymphocytes characterised by accumulation of small, mature-appearing lymphocytes in the blood, bone marrow and secondary lymphoid tissues. Presentation is heterogenous and the disease is often indolent and may not ever progress. Initiating treatment depends on symptoms and signs of disease progression.

Significant bone marrow failure with anaemia or thrombocytopenia, rapid doubling of lymphocyte count, rapidly progressing or symptomatic splenomegaly or adenopathy or significant systemic symptoms such as fatigue, weight loss and fever are among the indications for initiating treatment.[199,200]

49. Answer c

Pulmonary hypertension is a severe vascular disorder defined as mean pulmonary arterial pressure of 25mmHg or more at rest. Pulmonary arterial hypertension describes a subgroup with pulmonary arterial pressure of 25mmHg or greater as well as normal pulmonary capillary wedge pressure of 15mmHg or less and pulmonary vascular resistance of greater than 3 Wood units, and where other common causes of pulmonary hypertension such as chronic lung disease, chronic pulmonary thromboembolic disease or left heart failure are not present. Gold standard for measurement is with right heart catheterisation, although features such as signs of right ventricular overload may be apparent on echocardiogram. It may present with dyspnoea, reduced exercise tolerance, chest pain and fatigue or signs of right heart failure such as leg oedema. It is classified into five groups depending on its cause, and treatment varies depending on the cause:

I   pulmonary arterial hypertension

II   pulmonary hypertension due to left heart disease

III   pulmonary hypertension due to lung disease and/or hypoxaemia

IV   chronic thromboembolic pulmonary hypertension

V   pulmonary hypertension with unclear or multifactorial origin

Pulmonary arterial hypertension (group I) may be idiopathic, drug related or associated with connective tissue disease, portal hypertension, congenital cardiac malformations, hereditary haemorrhage telangiectasia and HIV infection. It may also be a heritable disease with mutations in the bone morphogenetic protein receptor 2 (BMPR2) found in 75% of patients in this grouping.[204,205]

50. Answer b

Wilson's disease can present with a variety of neuro ogical symptoms, often movement disorders such as tremor, dystonia, Parkinsonism and cerebellar manifestations. The most commonly described is dysarthria, reported in up to 97% of those with neurological manifestations of Wi son's disease.[208]

51. Answer d

Serum sodium measurements can be affected by serum glucose, protein and lipid levels. Pseudohyponatraemia occurs in settlings where serum protein or lipid levels are high, and direct measurement of serum osmolality may help to differentiate true hypotonicity or hyponatraemia from pseudohyponatraemia.

Hyponatraemia may occur in hyperglycaemia due to dilutional factors as water moves out of cells due to an increase in serum osmolality. However hyponatraemia may also occur due to osmotic diuresis occurring due to hyperglycaemia. As well as this, diabetes mellitus is associated with hyponatraemia even in the absence of hyperglycaemia. In general serum measurements of sodium should be corrected in those with hyperglycaemia by adding 1.6mmol/L to serum sodium for every 100mg/dL (5.5mmol/L) increment of glucose above normal up to 400mg/dL, and by adding 2.4mmol/L to serum sodium when serum glucose is higher than 400mg/dL (22.2mmol/L).

Endocrine causes of hyponatraemia such as hypopituitarism leading to adrenal dysfunction or primary adrenal insufficiency are not uncommon and should always be excluded. Hyponatraemia may occur in severe hypothyroidism but is less common.

Direct measurement of sodium levels with a direct potentiometer such as one of the most modern blood gas analysers can reliably measure true serum sodium concentration.[210]

52. Answer a

Chest x-ray changes in COVID-19 are quite variable. They are most commonly ground glass in appearance and affect the peripheral and low zones, but this is by no means uniform. Changes may be subtle and a normal chest x-ray does not exclude COVID-19 pneumonia.[212]

Lymphopenia is a typical feature of COVID-19.

Chilblain-like lesions on the hands and feet are a recognised sequela of COVID-19.[213]

Anosmia occurs in about half of those with COVID-19.[211]

53. Answer c

2015 EULAR-ACR recommendations for initial treatment of polymyalgia rheumatica recommend methotrexate as a steroid sparing agent in those with risk factors for relapse, prolonged therapy or adverse events related to steroids, or with insufficient response to steroids. The evidence for methotrexate in polymyalgia rheumatica has been mixed, but better than other DMARDs. The anti-interleukin 6 receptor tocilizumab has shown promise.[219,220,221]

54. Answer c

Postural tachycardia syndrome (POTS) is a syndrome characterised by chronic symptoms of orthostatic intolerance with sustained and excessive sinus tachycardia in the absence of orthostatic hypotension. Diagnosis depends on the chronicity of symptoms and the demonstration of a sustained increase in heart rate of 30 bpm or more within 10 minutes of standing in the absence of a postural drop in blood pressure.[222]

55. Answer a

Although there is not strong randomised-controlled evidence the first choice medical treatment for trigeminal neuralgia remains carbamazepine or oxcarbarbazepine.[224]

56. Answer d

Ultrasound features of a lymph node suggestive of malignancy are microcalcifications, peripheral vascularity, hyperechogenicity, rounded shape and cystic aspect.

Note the contrast with thyroid nodules where hypoechogenicity is a feature suggestive of malignancy.[228,229]

57. Answer d

Primary biliary cirrhosis (PBC) is an autoimmune disorder of the liver characterised by chronic biochemical cholestasis, positive anti-mitochondrial antibodies and liver histology showing nonsuppurative destructive cholangitis and interlobular bile duct destruction.

Anti-mitochondrial antibodies are positive in >90% of those with PBC. Most patients will have elevated aminotransferases. Raised immunoglobulins are common especially IgM. Treatment with ursodeoxycholic acid has been shown to improve survival and time to liver transplant.

The Mayo score is now used more than the Child-Pugh score to predict prognosis. It incorporates patients age, serum bilirubin, albumin, prothrombin time and degree of oedema.[232,233]

58. Answer e

Measurement of the QT interval is notoriously difficult. It is not the same on all ECG leads due to varying projections on different lead vector axes. Lead II is usually used to measure QT interval by convention.

If a U wave is present, it is not routinely included in the QT interval although this is controversial, as it does constitute part of cardiac repolarisation. Different methods have been tried to resolve this. In practice the largest wave in the TU wave complex is often measured.

Correction for heart rate is necessary to get an accurate QT interval. The Bazett formula is the oldest method and still the most commonly used ($QT_c=QT/RR^{1/2}$) but has limitations at lower and higher heart rates and other methods are available.

When measuring QT interval an average of three consecutive beats should be taken.

In 2005, a study of 877 physicians and cardiologists worldwide were asked to measure the QT interval of four relatively straighforward ECGs, with less than 25% getting all four correct when compared with a gold standard of 25 world experts. The authors concluded that the majority of physicians cannot recognise a long QT interval when they see one.[232,233]

59. Answer d

Clostridium difficile, a gram positive, anaerobic, spore-forming, toxin producing bacillus, was officially renamed Clostridioides difficile in 2016, to reflect differences between this species and other members of the clostridium genus. It has been known as a gut commensal for many years, and its association with diarrhoeal infection has increased since the introduction of antibiotics.

Age over 65 years increases the risk of clostridioides difficile infection (CDI) 10-fold. The risk of CDI increases 8 to 10 fold during antibiotic treatment and 4 weeks thereafter, and is still three fold higher for the next two months. Hospitalisation also increases the risk of CDI but community acquired infection is becoming more important, accounting for up to 30% of cases in some areas. The theory that gastric acid suppression may increase the risk of CDI has not been proven and it has been observed that gastric acid does not kill C difficile spores.

C difficile spores may survive in the environment for several months with toilets, furnishings, medical devices and mobile phones all potential reservoirs.[244]

60. Answer b

Upper extremity deep vein thromboses (UEDVT) accounts for 5% of all deep vein thrombosis. It may be primary or secondary. Primary UEDVT is usually associated with anatomical abnormalities causing venous compression as well as strenuous upper limb muscular effort. Secondary UEDVT is most commonly associated with malignancy or indwelling lines.

Wells score is a clinical probability tool used for lower limb DVT and is not useful in UEDVT. D Dimers can be useful to exclude the diagnosis in those with a low clinical probability, but imaging should be performed in all patients with suspected UEDVT with central venous catheter, pacemaker, patients with cancer, inpatients or those over 75 years of age. Ultrasound is the first line imaging modality and compares well with venogram, which is more invasive and involves radiation exposure. Anticoagulation is required for at least three months but may be required for longer in those with malignancy, indwelling lines or other provoking factors which cannot be resolved. Anticoagulation can be with low molecular weight heparin, vitamin K antagonists or direct oral anticoagulants.[245]

61. Answer d

Gastric antral vascular ectasia (GAVE) is also known as watermelon stomach and is characterised by its endoscopic 'watermelon' features of parallel red striped angiomatous lesions at antral mucosal folds. It is twice as common in females as compared to males. It is an acquired disorder of unknown aetiology. It can be associated with autoimmune disease such as systemic sclerosis, liver cirrhosis, cardiovascular disease and chronic renal failure. It may present with occult gastrointestinal blood loss leading to anaemia or overt gastrointestinal bleeding. 60-70% of those affected require repeated transfusions. No effective treatment has been established. There is some limited evidence that treatments such as corticosteroids may reduce anaemia occurrence, but no medical therapy is shown to normalise the characteristic endoscopic appearance.[246]

62. Answer a

Alzheimer's disease accounts for 60 to 80% of those presenting with dementia over the age of 65.[247]

63. Answer e

The HAS-BLED score estimates risk of bleeding on anticoagulation treatment. It gives a point for uncontrolled hypertension, renal disease, liver disease, stroke history, prior major bleeding or pred sposition to bleeding, labile INR, age>65 years, use of anti-platelet medication or NSAID and alcohol use.

Risk of falling is not in itself a risk of bleeding and it is estimated that a person would need to fall 295 times in one year for the benefits of warfarin therapy to be outweighed by the risk of intracranial haemorrhage. Anticoagulation should only be withheld in those in whom it is indicated if falls are severe and uncontrolled, such as seizures.[248]

64. Answer b

Herpes zoster (shingles) occurs due to reactivation of latent varicella zoster virus. Diagnosis is usually clinical, but where laboratory diagnosis is required VZV DNA PCR has the highest sensitivity and specificity and has become the gold standard. Antiviral treatment started within 72 hours of onset can reduce viral shedding and prevent new lesions, and should be considered even after 72 hours of onset in others, including the immunocompromised. Predictors for post herpetic neuralgia include the presence of prodromal symptoms, severity of pain, extent of rash, older age, immunosuppression, diabetes and the presence of zoster ophthalmicus. Corticosteroid treatment may help pain but does not shorten illness or reduce the incidence of post herpetic neuralgia. There is no evidence for the superiority of any one antiviral.[249]

65. Answer e

Bullous pemphigoid is the most common autoimmune bullous disorder. It occurs due to autoantibodies that target components of hemidesmosomes in the basement membrane zone. Classic bullous pemphigoid is more common in the elderly and the lesions are itchy. Non bullous presentations may occur.

Bullous pemphigoid creates a pro-thrombotic state with increased risk of venous thromboembolic disease and stroke during active disease.[250,251,252]

66. Answer a

The Kidney Disease Improving Global Outcome (KDIGO) organisation guidelines for diagnosis of acute kidney injury 2012 criteria are an increase in serum creatinine of 0.3mg/dL (26.53 µmol/L) in 48 hours, an increase in serum creatinine of at least 1.5 times baseline within the previous seven days, or urine volume below 0.5ml/kg/hour for six hours.[287]

67. Answer b

10 % of people will suffer a stroke within 90 days of a TIA or minor stroke. Aspirin therapy reduces this risk by 20%. Dual antiplatelet therapy was found to reduce this risk further in the POINT trial although at a cost of more bleeding events. Dual antiplatelet therapy is recommended in some guidelines within 24 hours after TIA or minor stroke.

The RESTART trial found that antiplatelet therapy was safe to use after haemorrhagic stroke in those with vascular disease, although it is not clear when it should be started. $ABCD_2$ score is often used to assess risk of stroke in those with TIA but is no longer felt to be a reliable indicator of risk.[253]

68. Answer a

Long term urate lowering treatment in gout is recommended in those with gout attacks once per year, or who have tophi, renal impairment, transplant-associated gout, nephrolithiasis or need diuretic treatment for heart failure. British and European guidelines recommend starting treatment 1-2 weeks after an acute attack but 2012 American guidelines support starting treatment during an acute attack.

Urate lowering treatment should be continued during an acute attack.[288]

69. Answer a

Bell's palsy is an idiopathic lower motor neurone palsy of CN VII. 29% have some permanent facial weakness, about half of these moderate to severe. Corticosteroids started early can reduce risk of permanent weakness, but there is conflicting evidence for antivirals. Palsy is thought to occur due to neural compression and facial nerve grafting surgery may help in those with persisting weakness if performed within 6 months

Lyme disease may present with facial weakness so all those with facial palsy should be tested for Lyme disease.[254]

70. Answer b

Current guidelines recommend corticosteroids for acute exacerbations of COPD should be continued for 5 days with no benefit seen in continuing treatment beyond 7 days.[255]

71. Answer d

The classification of chronic kidney disease is as follows:[275,276]

1	kidney damage with normal GFR	>90 ml/min/1.73m^2
2	kidney damage with mild decrease in GFR	60-89 ml/min/1.73m^2
3a	mild to moderate decrease in GFR	45-59 ml/min/1.73m^2
3b	moderate to severe decrease in GFR	30-44 ml/min/1.73m^2
4	severe decrease in GFR	15-29 ml/min/1.73m^2
5	end-stage renal disease	<15 ml/min/1.73m^2

72. Answer a

Up to 10% of those with DVT are subsequently diagnosed with a malignancy.[256]

73. Answer e

Autoimmune hepatitis is a chronic progressive liver disease characterised by high IgG levels, circulating autoantibodies, histological signs of hepatitis and a favourable response to immunosuppressive treatments. It is more common on women but does occur in men. Histological confirmation is required for diagnosis as many other typical findings such as hypergammaglobulinaemia, raised IgG levels and positive autoantibodies may not be present.[257]

74. Answer e

Familial hypercholesterolaemia is a common inherited condition resulting in prolonged exposure to high LDL levels and premature cardiovascular disease. In its most common form it is a monogenic autosomal dominant disorder affecting LDL receptors and therefore LDL uptake from the peripheral circulation. There is a gene dosage effect, in that homozygotes or compound heterozygotes have higher circulating LDL levels than those who are heterozygotes.[258]

75. Answer d

Focal motor seizures occur due to an epileptogenic lesion on the contralateral frontal lobe. Typically consciousness is not impaired. The seizure may take various forms.

Clonic seizures involve repeated short contractions of various muscle groups lasting less than 1 to 2 seconds, and are usually brief lasting 1 to 2 minutes.

Tonic seizures consist of sustained contractions of various muscle groups lasting more than 5 to 10 seconds resulting in posturing of the limbs and whole body.

Versive seizures involve sustained, forceful, involuntary turning of the head and eyes to one side due to tonic contraction of the head and eye muscles.

Tonic contractions in one hand progressing to clonic movements in the affected area, then with spread to the ipsilateral arm and to the ipsilateral foot and leg is known as a 'Jacksonian March'. It describes the seizure activity 'marching' from one affected area to other areas on the same side of the body.[259]

76. Answer c

Velcro rales refer to fine crackles audible on chest auscultation indicative of pulmonary fibrosis.[260]

77. Answer a

Darier disease is a rare autosomal dominant condition also known as keratosis follicularis. It is caused by a mutation in the ATP2A2 gene which encodes a calcium pump in the endoplasmic reticulum. This leads to aberrant junctional protein processing and poor cohesion between keratinocytes. Acantholysis, or the breakdown of connections between keratinocytes, is a feature. There is high penetrance but variable expressivity among those affected. Therefore most of those affected will have some manifestation but of highly variable severity. It is more frequent in men.

Mutations in the ATP2C1 gene cause Hailey-Hailey disease which also leads to aberrant junctional protein processing.[261]

78. Answer e

Complex regional pain syndrome (CRPS) is a chronic neurological condition occurring due to a traumatic insult. Clinical features include changes in skin temperature and colour, oedema, hyperalgesia and allodynia, with clinical features not occurring in a dermatomal distribution.[263]

79. Answer a

Benign paroxysmal positional vertigo (BPPV) is characterised by sudden, transitory vertigo sensation provoked by positional changes of the head with accompanying nystagmus. It is caused by aberrant signalling from the semicircular canals creating an illusion of motion. It is usually idiopathic but it may occur secondary to inner ear trauma or surgery, or secondary to inner ear conditions such as Meniere's disease, sudden sensorineural hearing loss or vestibular neuritis. The posterior semicircular canal is the most commonly affected, accounting for 80-90% of cases. If symptoms are triggered by turning to one side when lying flat, then that side is likely to be affected in posterior canal variant BPPV. Vertigo usually lasts less then 20 seconds. Hanging the head over the back if the bed on lying flat is not necessary when performing Dix-Hallpike maneuver.[263]

80. Answer c

Mixed connective tissue disease (MCTD) refers to a rheumatological overlap syndrome with clinical features of SLE, systemic sclerosis, polymyositis and rheumatoid arthritis. All of the above listed autoantibodies are associated with a particular overlap syndrome, of which there are a few. Anti-U1RNP antibodies are associated with MCTD.[264]

81. Answer c

Guillain Barre syndrome is a progressive motor weakness, usually symmetrical and beginning in the legs, and reaching its maximum weakness within four weeks of onset. It is assumed to be due to an immunological response to triggers such as surgery or infection. All of those listed are subtypes with acute inflammatory demyelinating polyneuropathy the most common presentation.[267,268]

82. Answer e

Ascending cholangitis, also known as acute cholangitis, is a bacterial infection of the extrahepatic biliary system. It is caused by biliary obstruction leading to bacteria 'ascending' from the duodenum into the common bile duct. Gallstones are the most frequent cause of ascending cholangitis. Cirrhosis is a risk factor for ascending cholangitis but not a cause.[269]

83. Answer d

Statin therapy is the cornerstone of dyslipidaemia treatment. Their benefit in reducing cardiovascular endpoints has been consistently shown. Lowering LDL-C levels by 2mmol/L has been associated with a reduction in cardiovascular events by 45%. The benefits of statins are distributed unevenly among populations, and the relative risk reduction needs to be interpreted in the context of an individual's underlying cardiovascular risk.[291]

84. Answer d

Autosomal dominant polycystic kidney disease (ADPKD) is associated with a fivefold increased risk of intracranial aneurysm (ICA). ICAs are detected in 8% of patients with ADPKD. The risk is further increased if there is a family history of ICA. Whether all patients with ADPKD should have presymptomatic screening for ICAs is controversial with no consensus, although some recommend screening for those with increased risk, especially if there is a family history of ICAs. Increased size, family history of ICAs, personal history of subarachnoid haemorrhage and posterior location of the ICA are all factors which increase risk of rupture.[270]

85. Answer a

Von Willebrand's disease is the most common inherited bleeding disorder.

It is characterised by mucosal bleeding and bleeding after surgery or trauma (although other types of bleeding also occur) and laboratory evidence of von Willebrand factor abnormalities, factor VIII abnormalities or both. Treatment is based on normalising von Willebrand factor and factor VIII levels using desmopressin or von Willebrand and factor VIII concentrate infusions.[270]

86. Answer c

The World Health Organisation and American Diabetes Association criteria for diagnosis of all types of diabetes mellitus are:

Fasting plasma glucose greater than or equal to 7.0 mmol/L (126mg/dL), or

2 hour plasma glucose of greater than or equal to 11.1mmol/L (200mg/dL) during an oral glucose tolerance test using a 75g glucose load, or

HbA1c greater than or equal to 6.5% (48mmol/mol), or

Random plasma glucose of greater than or equal to 11.1mmol/L (200mg/dL) in a symptomatic patient with classic hyperglycaemia symptoms

Where a state of hyperglycaemia is uncertain, two abnormal tests are required for diagnosis

HbA1c is not an appropriate test for diagnosing type 1 diabetes as the onset of hyperglycaemia may occur rapidly and may not be reflected in the result, and also there can be a delay in processing the test when compared to blood glucose levels.[273]

87. Answer a

Chronic kidney disease (CKD) is defined as a glomerular filtration rate (GFR) of <60ml/min of the presence of kidney damage for three months or more. Kidney damage can refer to pathological abnormalities documented by biopsy or imaging, protein-to-creatinine ratio of >200mg/g or albumin-to-creatinine ratio of >30 ml/min/1.73m^2, genetic renal disorder or history of renal transplantation. The majority of cases of CKD are progressive. Acute kidney injury increases the risk of developing chronic kidney disease. Duration, severity and frequency of episodes of acute kidney injury are seen as important factors in progression of chronic kidney disease. The principal cause of morbidity and mortality in those with chronic kidney disease is cardiovascular disease.

Renin-angiotensin-aldosterone system (RAAS) blockade is seen as an important strategy in CKD management. Single therapy with ACE inhibitors or angiotensin receptor blockers provides incomplete blockade. Studies with dual blockade have been disappointing. Although there have been reductions in proteinuria with dual blockade, there were increased risk of adverse outcomes and events.[275,276]

88. Answer d

A positive reaction in skin prick testing is a wheal of >3mm. A positive result may occur due to sensitisation and does not necessarily indicate allergy. Results are not always consistent with blood allergy testing such as RAST. It is useful in assessing any IgE-mediated allergy. There is a 0.077% risk of a serious systemic reaction during a skin prick test.[277]

89. Answer c

In COVID-1, serum IgM and IgA antibodies are secreted by days 5 to 7 after the onset of symptoms. IgG is secreted by days 7 to 10 after onset of symptoms.[279]

90. Answer d

Clinical and radiological findings in encephalitis may be non-specific and diagnosis of the cause of encephalitis may be difficult. Protein and WBC count on CSF analysis may be abnormal but again do not elucidate the cause. CSF analysis with PCR (polymerase chain reaction) is the most reliable way of diagnosing herpes simplex encephalitis. PCR is used to diagnose DNA viruses and reverse transcriptase PCR (RT-PCR) for RNA viruses.[280]

91. Answer b

Interferon-γ-release assays (IGRAs) such as the Quantiferon TB-Gold assay are used primarily to detect latent tuberculosis (TB). They offer an advantage over tuberculin skin testing (TST) in that they do not cross-react in those who have had previous BCG vaccination. They are also less likely

To cross-react with non-tuberculous mycobacteria (NTM) although there may be some cross-reaction with some NTM. They cannot distinguish between active and latent tuberculosis and are poorly predictive of who will progress from latent to active tuberculosis. IGRAs detect interferon-γ secretion by T lymphocytes which are stimulated by TB-specific antigens.[281,282,283]

92. Answer d

West Nile virus is a flavivirus spread by mosquitoes. 25% of those infected develop West Nile fever with a large variation in illness severity. <1% will develop neuroinvasive disease and this has a mortality rate of 10%. Older age is a risk factor for neuroinvasive disease. Significant prolonged functional difficulties are usual after neuroinvasive disease. Diagnosis is by detection of serum or cerebrospinal fluid IgM antibodies to West Nile virus.

Recent yellow fever or Japanese B encephalitis vaccination may produce a false positive serum antibody test.[284,285]

93. Answer d

Hepatitis E is an RNA virus and is a common infective agent worldwide. There are 8 known genotypes. Genotypes 1-4 are the most frequently described in humans. Most infections are asymptomatic but acute liver failure or acute on chronic liver failure may occur.

Genotypes 1 and 2 cause frequent infections through contaminated drinking water in the tropics. No zoonotic reservoir has been identified. Pregnant women are especially vulnerable to acute liver failure secondary to infection with genotype 1.

Genotypes 3 and 4 are zoonotic infections with pigs the main reservoir. These genotypes are associated with a less severe illness than genotypes 1 and 2, however are associated with an increased risk of acute on chronic liver failure in those with underlying liver disease.

A recombinant hepatitis E vaccine has been approved for use in China.[286]

94. Answer c

The Kidney Disease Improving Global Outcome (KDIGO) organisation guidelines for diagnosis of acute kidney injury 2012 criteria are an increase in serum creatinine of 0.3mg/dL (26.53 µmol/L) in 48 hours, an increase in serum creatinine of at least 1.5 times baseline within the previous seven days, or urine volume below 0.5ml/kg/hour for six hours.[287]

95. Answer e

Gout is the most common inflammatory arthropathy and occurs due to hyperuricaemia and monosodium crystal deposition. It is usually a clinical diagnosis although joint aspiration can be used to aid diagnosis where doubt exists. Negatively birefringent needle-shaped monosodium urate crystals are seen on polarised light microscopy. Raised white bloods cells and inflammatory markers are common in acute gout. Serum uric acid is often reduced during an attack and should be checked 1-2 weeks after resolution.

Statins and macrolides interact with colchicine potentially increasing the risk of colchicine toxicity.[288]

96. Answer d

Posterior circulation stroke occurs due occlusion of part of the vertebrobasilar arterial system affecting areas of the brain such as the brain stem, cerebellum, midbrain, thalamuses and occipital cortex. It may be more difficult to diagnose than anterior circulation stroke and can present with subtle visual or balance problems. Hemiparesis may occur in anterior or posterior circulation stroke. FAST score (The prehospital Face Arm Speech Test) has a lower sensitivity in posterior circulation stroke than anterior circulation stroke. CT scan has lower sensitivity for posterior circulation stroke than anterior circulation stroke and MRI is preferred if available. Tissue plasminogen activator can be used within 4.5 hours.

Risk of stroke after posterior circulation stroke is at least as high as anterior circulation stroke.[289]

97. Answer d

Fabry disease is an x-linked lysosomal storage disorder caused by mutations to the GLA gene resulting in abnormal activity of the α-galactosidase A enzyme. This leads to accumulation of glycolipids in a range of organs throughout the body. Different GLA mutations may lead to varying levels of α-galactosidase A. Severity of clinical phenotype can vary significantly even among family members with the same GLA mutation. Classic Fabry disease presents in male children with severe neuropathic pain, skin abnormalities such as angiokeratomas, abdominal pain and bloating. Progressive renal impairment and cardiac complications such as left ventricular hypertrophy, myocardial fibrosis and arrhythmias develop. Stroke, TIAs and premature death occur.

A less severe adult phenotype also exists in males. Affected females can vary from no symptoms to a severe form of the disease.

Demonstration of normal levels of the affected enzyme α-galactosidase A are sufficient to exclude the diagnosis in males but not in females where measured levels may be normal. Genetic testing or tissue biopsy of affected organs may be necessary. Enzyme levels can be measured in plasma, leukocytes or dried blood spot.

Enzyme replacement therapy is the cornerstone of treatment and is given every two weeks by intravenous infusion.[290]

98. Answer a

Some evidence exists that fibrates have a modest effect on reducing cardiovascular events, especially non-fatal myocardial infarction, there is no evidence that they reduce cardiovascular or all-cause mortality in primary or secondary prevention. Any benefits in reducing cardiovascular events tend to disappear when combined with statin treatment. Clofibrate, the earliest fibrate, was withdrawn in 2002 when it was found to increase all-cause mortality in a large primary prevention study. Fibrates have fallen out of favour in most guidelines for treatment of dyslipidaemia, although may be considered in severe hypertriglyceridemia in particular where pancreatitis is a risk.[291]

99. Answer e

Latent autoimmune diabetes of adulthood (LADA) is defined by three criteria:

- Onset at over 30 years of age

- Presence of at least one circulating autoantibody associated with type 1 diabetes mellitus

- Initial insulin independence (within the first 6 months)

It is an indolent type of type 1 diabetes often mistaken for type 2 diabetes. Beta cell destruction occurs resulting in requirement for insulin and potential for ketoacidosis.[293]

100. Answer d

Chikungunya is an arboviral infection with a clinical presentation similar to Dengue fever with some important differences. Retro-orbital headache which is a common feature of Dengue fever is conspicuously absent in Chikungunya.[295]

1. The most common form of primary glomerulonephritis worldwide is:
   a. IgA nephropathy
   b. Anti-glomerular basement membrane disease
   c. Minimal-change disease
   d. Membranous nephropathy
   e. Focal segmental glomerulosclerosis

2. Löfgren syndrome:
   a. Has a poor prognosis with progressively worsening respiratory symptoms
   b. Biopsy of the erythema nodosum rash shows features which differentiate it from erythema nodosum from other causes
   c. Arthritis is not a feature
   d. Requires histological confirmation of non-caseating granulomas for diagnosis
   e. Requires chest radiology for diagnosis

3. Heart failure with preserved ejection fraction (HFpEF):
   a. Occurs due to impaired left ventricular relaxation and filling
   b. Is defined as heart failure with ejection fraction > 40%
   c. Is more common than heart failure with reduced ejection fraction (HFrEF)
   d. HFpEF has a distinct clinical presentation to HFrEF
   e. Brain-type natriuretic peptide (BNP) measurement is not helpful in HFpEF

4. Coronaviruses:
   a. Are DNA viruses
   b. May cause illness with a mortality up to 36%
   c. Affect only humans
   d. Mainly cause gastrointestinal infections
   e. Are commonly associated with lymphocytosis

5. Hepatocyte nuclear factor 1α (HNF1A) and hepatocyte nuclear factor 4α (HNF4A) maturity onset diabetes:
   - a. Result in stable long-term asymptomatic hyperglycaemia
   - b. Do not require treatment
   - c. Do not lead to long term microvascular complications
   - d. Respond well to sulphonylurea medication
   - e. Are associated with insulin resistance

6. Bicuspid aortic valve with no other aortic valve or ascending aorta abnormalities should have surveillance with transthoracic echocardiogram every:
   - a. 1-2 years
   - b. 2-3 years
   - c. 4-5 years
   - d. 5-10 years
   - e. No surveillance is needed

7. Anti-retroviral treatment in HIV-positive patients:
   - a. Should be deferred until CD4+ counts have dropped to 350 cells per cubic millimetre
   - b. Should be offered to all patients with HIV
   - c. Will not reduce an individual's infectivity
   - d. Excludes the possibility of developing AIDS
   - e. Compliance to treatment does not affect resistance

8. Decompensated liver disease:
   - a. The most common complication is gastrointestinal bleeding
   - b. Blood transfusion for gastrointestinal bleeding in those with decompensated liver disease may increase rebleeding and mortality
   - c. A raised serum ammonia level in a jaundiced patient is diagnostic of hepatic encephalopathy
   - d. Patients should aim for 6 soft bowel motions per day using laxatives
   - e. High volumes of 0.9% saline and 5% dextrose should be used if the patient is hypovolaemic

9. Which of the following are not useful criteria in the diagnosis of Marfan syndrome:
    a.   High-arched palate
    b.   Family history
    c.   Aortic root disease
    d.   Ectopia lentis
    e.   Fibrillin 1 (FBN1) gene mutation

10. Correct performance of spirometry involves:
    a.   Coughing forcefully into the mouthpiece
    b.   Breathing in fully, then placing the mouth around the mouthpiece and breathing out fully, then breathing in maximally again
    c.   Breathing out fully, then placing mouth around the mouthpiece and breathing in fully and then out again
    d.   Taking a short breath in and then breathing out fully
    e.   Taking a short breath out and then inspiring maximally

11. Aortic stenosis:
    a.   Is most commonly congenital
    b.   Is more common in those under than over 70 years of age
    c.   In younger patients bicuspid aortic valve is the most common cause
    d.   Prognosis is good even in untreated symptomatic patients
    e.   The outcome of surgical aortic valve replacement is poor in the elderly

12. Adrenal crisis arises due to an absolute deficiency of:
    a.   ACTH
    b.   Renin
    c.   Cortisol
    d.   Aldosterone
    e.   ADH

13. Lung nodules:
    a. The largest of multiple nodules can be assumed to be the malignant one
    b. Are more likely to be malignant in the lower lobes
    c. Calcification of a nodule indicates that it is likely to be malignant
    d. Fat attenuation of a nodule indicates that it is likely to be malignant
    e. Size and growth rate are the most important imaging factors indicating likely malignancy of a lung nodule

14. Polymerase chain reaction (PCR) for virus testing:
    a. Is less commonly used for detecting viruses than viral culture
    b. Samples must be tested within 24 hours of collection
    c. Has high sensitivity and specificity
    d. Detects only live virus
    e. A positive test indicates that the subject remains infectious

15. The most common inherited cause of aplastic anaemia is:
    a. Seckel syndrome
    b. Fanconi anaemia
    c. Dyskeratosis congenita
    d. Diamond-Blackfan syndrome
    e. Bloom syndrome

16. Stevens-Johnson syndrome/toxic epidermal necrolysis (SJS/TEN):
    a. Is characterised by partial-thickness epidermal necrolysis
    b. Mucosal symptoms always precede systemic symptoms
    c. Is caused more often by infection than by medication
    d. Corticosteroid use is the most important intervention
    e. Progression from SJS to TEN depends on percentage of body surface area involvement

17. Penicillin allergy:
    a. Cross reactivity between penicillin and cephalosporin allergy is usually due to the shared betalactam ring
    b. Occurs only as an immediate hypersensitivity reaction rather than as a delayed hypersensitivity reaction
    c. A childhood reaction to penicillin is likely to be a true penicillin allergy
    d. Cefalexin can be safely used in true penicillin allergy without further assessment
    e. Is associated with an increased risk of clostridium difficile infection

18. The incidence of which of the following adverse effects of methotrexate can be reduced by folate supplementation:
    a. Pulmonary fibrosis
    b. Skin nodulosis
    c. Fatigue
    d. Cytopenias
    e. Renal toxicity

19. Primary ciliary dyskinesia (PCD):
    a. Is an autosomal dominant condition
    b. May be associated with asplenia
    c. Adult onset respiratory symptoms are typical
    d. Female reproductive difficulties do not occur
    e. All affected men are infertile

20. Which of the following does not confer increased risk of stroke in atrial fibrillation:
    a. Male gender
    b. Obstructive sleep apnoea
    c. Heart failure with preserved ejection fraction
    d. Controlled hypertension
    e. Age > 65

21. The most common extranodal presentation of non-Hodgkins lymphoma is:
   a.   Gastrointestinal
   b.   Cutaneous
   c.   Pulmonary
   d.   Intracranial
   e.   Cardiac

22. Coeliac disease:
   a.   The malabsorption syndrome of diarrhoea, weight loss and asthenia presents more commonly in adults than in children
   b.   Macrocytic anaemia is a more common presentation than microcytic anaemia in coeliac disease
   c.   Is associated with HLA antigens DQ2 and DQ8
   d.   A gluten-free diet will not affect elevated liver transaminases in coeliac disease
   e.   Thrombocytopenia may be a sign of hyposplenism

23. Acromegaly:
   a.   Densely granulated somatroph adenomas are more aggressive
   b.   Does not require surgical adenoma resection
   c.   Elevated morning growth hormone levels may be sufficient for diagnosis
   d.   Hypertension will resolve after treatment of acromegaly
   e.   30% will get gastrointestinal side effects on treatment with somatropin ligand treatment

24. If a Weber test lateralises to one side this indicates:
   a.   A contralateral conductive hearing loss
   b.   An ipsilateral conductive hearing loss
   c.   An ipsilateral sensorineural hearing loss
   d.   Normal hearing
   e.   Noise-induced hearing loss

25. Thalidomide syndrome:

a. Facial disfigurement is the most common feature
b. Does not cause any internal organ derangement
c. Phocomelia refers to visual impairment resulting from thalidomide exposure
d. The most common long-term complication is increased cardiovascular risk
e. Is associated with an increased risk of osteoarthritis compared with the general population

26. Cushing disease:

a. Is the same as Cushing syndrome
b. May occur due to prolonged exogenous steroid use
c. Can be diagnosed with an MRI scan
d. Is more likely to present with mass effects from a pituitary adenoma than biochemical effects of excess hormone production
e. Is best treated surgically

27. Chronic atrophic gastritis:

a. Is not a pre-malignant condition
b. May present with depression
c. Is best diagnosed serologically
d. It is straightforward to distinguish whether it is caused by Helicobacter pylori infection or an autoimmune cause
e. Associated vitamin B12 deficiency does not progress to neurological complications

28. Hidradenitis suppurativa:

a. Is not more common if there is a family history
b. Is caused by anaerobic and not by aerobic bacteria
c. Does not response to antibiotic treatment
d. Biologic disease-modifying antirheumatic drugs (DMARDs) have a role in treatment
e. Is more common in men

29. Primary hyperparathyroidism:
    a.   Parathyroid imaging is needed for diagnosis
    b.   Vitamin D supplementation should not be given
    c.   Serum calcium is always raised
    d.   Will eventually require surgery in all cases
    e.   Most commonly arises from a single parathyroid adenoma

30. The Vaughan Williams class of atenolol is:
    a.   IA
    b.   IC
    c.   II
    d.   III
    e.   IV

31. Bechet's disease:
    a.   Only occurs in those who are HLA B27 positive
    b.   Requires raised inflammatory markers for diagnosis
    c.   Commonly affects the kidneys
    d.   Is most common along the Silk Road
    e.   Oral ulceration is uncommon

32. The most common mutation leading to hereditary haemochromatosis is:
    a.   C282Y homozygous
    b.   H63D homozygous
    c.   C282Y/H63D compound heterozygous
    d.   S65C homozygous
    e.   C282Y heterozygous

33. Epworth sleepiness scale in obstructive sleep apnoea (OSA):
    a.   Is a useful screening tool for OSA
    b.   Will have a higher score with reduced daytime sleepiness
    c.   Has a high sensitivity and specificity for OSA diagnosis
    d.   Daytime sleepiness is considered severe if score is greater than 10
    e.   May not be reliable due to potential secondary gain

34. Thyroid dysfunction and cardiovascular risk:
    a.   Hyperthyroidism reduces cholesterol levels
    b.   Hypothyroidism reduces LDL levels
    c.   Overt hyperthyroidism reduces cardiovascular mortality
    d.   Over hyperthyroidism reduces stroke risk
    e.   Subclinical hyperthyroidism is associated with increased cardiovascular risk

35. D Dimer testing is useful:
    a.   To predict stroke risk in individuals with atrial fibrillation
    b.   To predict cardiovascular risk in individuals with HIV infection
    c.   In predicting mortality in those with cardiovascular disease
    d.   In identifying hospitalised medically ill patients who may have increased risk of venous thromboembolic disease
    e.   In diagnosing acute coronary syndrome in individuals with chest pain

36. Ebola virus disease:
    a.   Most affected individuals will have haemorrhagic complications
    b.   Serology is the most common method used for diagnosis
    c.   No vaccine is available
    d.   Contacts of a case need to be followed up for 21 days as part of disease control measures
    e.   No antiviral treatment exists

37. Which of the following confers increased risk of developing ulcerative colitis:
    a. Breast feeding
    b. Previous appendicectomy
    c. Active smoking
    d. Non steroidal anti-inflammatory medication use
    e. Antibiotic use

38. Which of the following is not one of the minor criteria on the Duke Modified Criteria for diagnosis of infective endocarditis:
    a. Predisposing cardiac condition
    b. Intravenous drug use
    c. Intracranial haemorrhage
    d. Septic pulmonary emboli
    e. New valvular regurgitation

39. Metformin associated lactic acidosis:
    a. Of the biguanides, lactic acidosis occurs most frequently with metformin
    b. Will not occur with usual doses of metformin
    c. Is most likely to occur in those with relatively high circulating levels of metformin above 5mcg/ml
    d. Is rarely fatal
    e. Will not occur in those with mild renal dysfunction

40. Milder forms of alpha thalassaemia may be misdiagnosed as:
    a. Iron deficiency
    b. Folic acid deficiency
    c. Vitamin B12 deficiency
    d. Multiple myeloma
    e. Anaemia of chronic disease

41. Which of the following is the most effective treatment to reduce risk of recurrent stroke after a noncardioembolic ischaemic stroke:
    a.   Aspirin alone
    b.   Clopidogrel alone
    c.   Aspirin and clopidogrel combined
    d.   Warfarin
    e.   Direct oral anticoagulant

42. The negative predictive value of a test refers to:
    a.   The proportion of people with a condition who have a positive test result
    b.   The proportion of people without a condition who have a negative test result
    c.   The proportion of people with a condition with a given test result (either positive or negative) divided by the proportion of people without the condition with that result
    d.   The post-test probability that a person with a positive test result has the condition
    e.   The post-test probability that a person with a negative test result does not have the condition

43. Which of the following does <u>not</u> occur in tumour lysis syndrome:
    a.   Hyperkalaemia
    b.   Hyperuricaemia
    c.   Hypocalcaemia
    d.   Hypokalaemia
    e.   Hyperphosphataemia

44. Membranous nephropathy:
    a.   May be associated with underlying malignancy
    b.   Is more likely to be secondary rather than primary in adults than in children
    c.   Specific antibodies against podocyte antigens are not useful prognostic indicators
    d.   Angiotensin II blockade is likely to eliminate proteinuria even in those with nephrotic syndrome
    e.   Progression to end-stage renal failure is uncommon

45. Which of the following is the most useful clinical sign in the diagnosis of hypersensitivity pneumonitis:
    a.   Digital clubbing
    b.   Inspiratory crackles on lung auscultation
    c.   Expiratory wheeze on lung auscultation
    d.   Tachypnoea
    e.   Persistent cough

46. The most common psychiatric manifestation of Wilson's disease is:
    a.   Psychosis
    b.   Personality disorder
    c.   Behavioural disorder
    d.   Depression
    e.   Catatonia

47. Psoriasis:
    a.   Plaques involve only the epidermal layer of the skin
    b.   80% of those affected will develop psoriatic arthropathy
    c.   Nails will be affected in over half of patients with psoriasis
    d.   Nail involvement is less common in those with psoriatic arthropathy than those with skin involvement only
    e.   Nail involvement will not occur without skin involvement

48. Bisphosphonates reduce hip fracture risk by:
    a.   5-10%
    b.   10-20%
    c.   30-40%
    d.   40-50%
    e.   80-90%

49. Type 1 diabetes:
    a. Obesity is a risk factor for its development
    b. Most individuals achieve recommended Hb A1 targets
    c. Hypoglycaemic events cause more deaths than diabetic ketoacidosis in those with type 1 diabetes
    d. Microvascular complications will manifest only as retinopathy, neuropathy or nephropathy.
    e. Microvascular complications are the major cause of premature morbidity and mortality

50. Which of the following is not associated with increased risk of disease progression to cirrhosis in chronic hepatitis C infection:
    a. Developing infection under age 40 years
    b. Male gender
    c. Coinfection with hepatitis B virus
    d. Coinfection with HIV
    e. Alcohol consumption greater than 50g per day

51. Which of the following are not one of the ACR-EULAR criteria for the diagnosis of rheumatoid arthritis:
    a. Symmetric polyarthritis
    b. Positive rheumatoid factor
    c. Positive anti-citrullinated protein antibodies
    d. Clinical synovitis of one joint
    e. Abnormal CRP

52. The most commonly documented drug allergy is to:
    a. Penicillin
    b. Cephalosporins
    c. Macrolides
    d. Quinolones
    e. Sulphonamides

53. Lithium treatment and thyroid dysfunction:
    a.   Most commonly manifests as overt hypothyroidism
    b.   The presence of antithyroid antibodies increases the risk of developing thyroid dysfunction secondary to lithium treatment
    c.   Can be diagnosed clinically
    d.   Goitre is not a feature
    e.   Lithium should be stopped when thyroid dysfunction occurs

54. Subacute combined immunodeficiency (SCID):
    a.   Is rarely fatal
    b.   Affects only B lymphocytes and not T lymphocytes
    c.   Presents usually as repeated bacterial infections in adults
    d.   Can be screened for with an assay to detect T cell receptor excision c rcle
    e.   No treatments are available

55. The most common form of congenital heart disease occurring in Down syndrome is:
    a.   Atrial septal defect
    b.   Ventricular septal defect
    c.   Secundum atrial septal defect
    d.   Tetralogy of Fallot
    e.   Patent ductus arteriosus

56. Which of the following is most likely to be useful in reducing the risk of transfusion-associated circulatory overload (TACO) after blood product transfusion:
    a.   Pooling blood products from multiple donors
    b.   Screening blood products for antibodies
    c.   Using male-only blood donated products
    d.   Screening blood products for blood borne viruses
    e.   Pre-transfusion diuresis

57. Trousseau's signs is carpopedal spasm after inflation of a sphygmomanometer above the systolic blood pressure and is seen in:
   a. Hypocalcaemia
   b. Hypercalcaemia
   c. Hyperkalaemia
   d. Hypokalaemia
   e. Hyponatraemia

58. In acute unilateral facial palsy, which of the following suggests an alternative diagnosis to Bells palsy:
   a. Absence of pain
   b. Sparing of forehead muscles
   c. Involvement of forehead muscles
   d. Normal ear examination
   e. Partial facial paralysis only

59. Water deprivation test:
   a. Can be performed at home
   b. Is not helpful in diagnosing primary polydipsia
   c. Urine output will fall in diabetes insipidus
   d. Urine osmolality will remain less than 750mOsm/kg in a patient with diabetes insipidus
   e. Patients with nephrogenic diabetes insipidus will not respond to desmopressin during the test

60. Sticky platelet syndrome:
   a. Is an acquired thrombophilia
   b. Predisposes to venous thromboembolism only
   c. Predisposes to arterial thrombosis only
   d. Is associated with increased risk of migraine with aura
   e. Is not associated with pregnancy complications

61. Porphyria cutanea tarda (PCT):
a. Most commonly presents with neurological symptoms
b. Usually presents initially in childhood
c. Iron deficiency can worsen symptoms
d. Phlebotomy is an effective treatment
e. Skin rash tends to occur in sun protected areas

62. Paget's disease of bone:
a. May be cured after a single bisphosphonate infusion
b. Lesions show signs of inflammation histologically
c. Radionuclide scans are better than plain x ray for diagnosis
d. Lesions affect axial skeleton only
e. Lesions can migrate spontaneously to adjacent bones

63. Rabies:
a. Results only from dog bites
b. Always leads to paralysis
c. Previous immunisation does not affect treatment
d. Post exposure vaccination is not useful
e. Death is inevitable once symptoms appear

64. Cimex lectularis:
a. Are the common bedbug
b. Cause scabies
c. Are head lice
d. Cause Lyme disease
e. Cause Orf

65. Hyperthyroidism:

    a.   Atrial fibrillation secondary to hyperthyroidism is more likely to cause stroke than atrial fibrillation without associated hyperthyroidism

    b.   Radioactive iodine uptake by the thyroid gland is not increased in true hyperthyroidism

    c.   Radioactive iodine uptake by the thyroid gland is increased in those with thyrotoxicosis from exogenous sources of thyroid hormone

    d.   Antithyroid drugs should not be used in Graves' disease as it rarely goes into remission

    e.   Propylthiouracil should not be used in pregnancy

66. Kimmelstiel-Wilson nodules are:

    a.   Renal nodular lesions associated with diabetic glomerulosclerosis

    b.   Renal nodular lesions associated with hypertensive nephropathy

    c.   Renal nodular lesions associated with minimal change disease

    d.   Renal nodular lesions associated with crescentic glomerulonephritis

    e.   Renal nodular lesions associated with membranous glomerulonephritis

67. Which of the following is more likely to lead to type 1 respiratory failure rather than type 2 respiratory failure:

    a.   Neuromuscular disease

    b.   Opiate toxicity

    c.   Obesity

    d.   Severe COVID-19

    e.   Over-oxygenation

68. The most common cause of secondary hypertension is:

    a.   Phaeochromocytoma

    b.   Cushing's syndrome

    c.   Primary aldosteronism

    d.   Polycystic kidney disease

    e.   Hyperparathyroidism

69. The first medication shown to reduce mortality in COVID 19 was:

a. Dexamethasone
b. Remdesivir
c. Hydroxychloroquine
d. Lopinavir
e. Ritonavir

70. The spine:

a. Intervertebral disks have a rich vascular supply
b. Biomechanical loads are predom nantly borne by the nucleus pulposus
c. Disk herniation involves herniation of the annulus fibrosis
d. End plate calcification will not affect disk homeostasis
e. Cervical disks are not sensitive to pain

71. Chronic lymphocytic leukaemia (CLL):

a. Patients with mutated IGHV CLL have more aggressive disease than unmutated IGHV CLL
b. Can be transmitted by blood transfusion
c. Deletion in chromosome 13q14.3 (del(13q)) occurs in a minority of patients with CLL and is associated with a poor prognosis
d. Is the most common adult leukaemia in western countries
e. Incidence decreases with increasing age

72. Lung cancer staging:

a. Is relevant only for non-small cell lung cancer
b. Is not affected by primary tumour size
c. Carcinoma in situ is included in staging classification
d. Stage I to IIIa non-small cell lung cancer are potentially curative with surgical resection
e. CT scan is the most sensitive modality for identifying mediastinal metastases

73. Pulmonary hypertension:
    a.   Calcium channel blockers are indicated in certain circumstances
    b.   All patients should be treated with anticoagulation
    c.   All patients will require oxygen
    d.   All patients will require treatment with loop diuretics
    e.   Exercise should be discouraged

74. The most common form of bleeding in hereditary haemorrhagic telangiectasia is:
    a.   Malena
    b.   Bright red rectal bleeding
    c.   Haematuria
    d.   Epistaxis
    e.   Haemoptysis

75. Mesothelioma:
    a.   Is not always associated with a history of asbestos exposure
    b.   Is associated with a latency period of 10 years following asbestos exposure
    c.   Is most commonly associated with exposure to serpentine (chrysotile) asbestos fibres
    d.   Has been associated with human papilloma virus
    e.   The pericardium is the most common site involved after the pleura

76. Kayser-Fleischer rings in Wilson's disease:
    a.   Are rare in those with neurological manifestations of Wilson's disease
    b.   Are unrelated to copper accumulation
    c.   Does not require slit lamp examination for diagnosis
    d.   Similar changes may be seen in primary biliary cirrhosis and myeloma
    e.   Are always green in colour

77. Diabetes insipidus is unlikely if 24 hour urinary volume is less than:
    a.   0.5litres
    b.   1.5litres
    c.   2.5litres
    d.   3.5litres
    e.   4.5litres

78. Anosmia:
    a.   When caused by COVID-19 is likely to improve with oral corticosteroids
    b.   When caused by COVID-19 is likely be permanent
    c.   When caused by COVID-19 is always accompanied by other symptoms
    d.   Occurs in about half of those with COVID-19
    e.   When caused by COVID-19 taste will not be affected

79. Faecal microbiota transplantation:
    a.   Is less effective than vancomycin in treating clostridioides difficile infection
    b.   Cannot be given orally
    c.   Potential donors do not need to be screened for infection
    d.   Donated samples may be frozen
    e.   Can be delivered only via colonoscopic transfer

80. Bacillus Calmette-Guerin (BCG) vaccination:
    a.   Can be safely given in the immunosuppressed
    b.   Is more effective in adults than in children
    c.   Will not cause disseminated infection
    d.   Should be given to all healthcare workers
    e.   Can be administered intravesically in the treatment of bladder cancer

81. Which of the following is the least common predisposing factor to native valve endocarditis in developed countries:
    a. Intravenous drug use
    b. Rheumatic heart disease
    c. Intracardiac devices
    d. Degenerative valvular disease
    e. Congenital heart disease

82. Initial corticosteroid treatment for polymyalgia rheumatica should be:
    a. Oral prednisolone 5-10mg per day
    b. Oral prednisolone 12.5-25mg per day
    c. Oral prednisolone 25-35mg per day
    d. Oral prednisolone 35-50mg per day
    e. Oral prednisolone 50-60mg per day

83. Which of the following is not a factor associated with postural tachycardia syndrome:
    a. Joint hypermobility
    b. Female gender
    c. Dependent acrocyanosis
    d. Resolution of symptoms with cardiac ablation
    e. Fibromyalgia

84. Ehlers Danlos syndrome:
    a. Is divided into several subtypes
    b. Is primarily a condition caused by abnormalities in elastin fibres
    c. Skin fragility is not a feature
    d. Is diagnosed using the Brighton criteria
    e. Is never life threatening

85. Trigeminal neuralgia:

 a. Is most commonly idiopathic
 b. Is most commonly caused by intracranial vascular compression of the trigeminal nerve root
 c. Is most commonly caused by multiple sclerosis
 d. Is most commonly caused by a benign cerebellopontine angle tumour
 e. Is most commonly caused by a malignant brain tumour

86. Post-acute COVID-19:

 a. Requires a positive COVID-19 test for diagnosis
 b. Only occurs in those who have had severe COVID-19
 c. The most common symptoms are headaches, lightheadedness and dyspnoea
 d. Occurs in 90% of those who have had COVID-19
 e. Psychological manifestation such as anxiety can be a feature

87. Ishihara's test:

 a. Is not useful for identifying red-green colour vision deficiency
 b. Can detect reduced blue colour vision deficiency
 c. Has been shown to be highly sensitive and specific
 d. Is available only in 24-plate editions
 e. Can provide an assessment of severity of colour vision deficiency

88. Thyroid nodules:

 a. When detected incidentally on CT, most do not require dedicated ultrasound
 b. Nodules wider than they are tall on ultrasound are more likely to be malignant than nodules taller than they are wide
 c. Hyperfunctioning nodules are more likely to be malignant than non-functioning nodules
 d. Surgical intervention should be considered for nodules >4cm diameter even with benign cytology
 e. Core needle biopsy is preferred to fine needle aspirate for obtaining a tissue diagnosis

89. Anti-mitochondrial antibodies:
    a. Are detected in 50% of those with primary biliary cirrhosis
    b. Are detected in 10% of the general population
    c. Are detected in 8% of those with hepatitis C infection
    d. Of those in the general population with positive anti-mitochondrial antibodies without primary biliary cirrhosis, all will subsequently develop the condition
    e. In those in the general population with positive anti-mitochondrial antibodies without primary biliary cirrhosis, liver monitoring is not required

90. In 1957 a family was described in which four of six children had recurring fainting episodes and deafness. Three of the children died in childhood. Pre-mortem and post mortem investigations were normal except for a prolonged QT interval on ECG. What was the diagnosis:
    a. Wolf Parkinson White syndrome
    b. Jervell Lange Nielson syndrome
    c. Romano Ward syndrome
    d. Brugada syndrome
    e. Arrhythmogenic right ventricular cardiomyopathy

91. Gabapentinoids (gabapentin and pregabalin):
    a. Were originally developed as analgesics
    b. Gabapentin is more potent in its receptor binding than pregabalin
    c. Gabapentin has higher bioavailability than pregabalin
    d. Are useful in the prophylaxis of migraine
    e. Caution should be used in initiating these medications in those with a history of addiction

92. Clostriodioides difficile infection (CDI):
    a. Is the most common cause of nosocomial diarrhoea
    b. Is more common in nursing home residents than in those in acute hospitals
    c. Is more common in those on proton pump inhibitors
    d. Rarely occurs due to spore transmission
    e. Is rarely found as a commensal in children

93. Alzheimer's disease:

a. Biomarkers are not useful in diagnosis
b. Visuospatial awareness is never affected
c. A negative amyloid PET scan strongly suggests another diagnosis
d. Cerebrospinal fluid may show an increase in CSF amyloid β
e. The first step in treatment after diagnosis is to start a cholinesterase inhibitor

94. Anticoagulation:

a. Direct oral anticoagulants (DOACs) are less effective than warfarin at reducing stroke in those with atrial fibrillation
b. All cause mortality is increased in those on DOACs versus warfarin in those with atrial fibrillation
c. DOACs have a higher risk of major bleeding than warfarin
d. DOACs have a higher risk of intracranial bleeding than warfarin
e. The risk of gastrointestinal bleeding is higher with some DOACs than with warfarin

95. Nikolsky's sign:

a. Describes the appearance of a rash on an area of skin trauma
b. Is positive in bullous pemphigoid
c. Is negative in pemphigus
d. Reflects skin acantholysis
e. Will be positive only on skin affected by rash

96. Familial hypercholesterolaemia:

a. Is rare
b. Premature cardiovascular disease will not affect heterozygotes
c. Statin use may be indicated in children with familial hypercholesterolaemia
d. Absence of typical genetic mutations excludes the diagnosis
e. Risk scores such as the Framingham Risk Score are useful in those with familial hypercholesterolaemia

97. Pulmonary fibrosis:
    a.   Is progressive in all patients
    b.   Serological markers are useful to assess disease progression
    c.   Supplemental oxygen is not indicated
    d.   Pulmonary rehabilitation has been shown to improve symptoms and quality of life
    e.   Immunosuppressive treatments are useful in all patients

98. Guillain Barre syndrome:
    a.   10% of patients will die
    b.   Corticosteroids speed time to recovery
    c.   Has been described after SARS CoV2 infection
    d.   Intravenous immunoglobulin is of no benefit
    e.   5% will require mechanical ventilation

99. Latent tuberculosis:
    a.   There will be a negative tuberculin skin test
    b.   There will be a negative Interferon-γ-release assay test
    c.   The highest risk time for transformation to active tuberculosis is 5-10 years after initial infection
    d.   Is contagious
    e.   Risk of progression to active TB is 20 times higher in those with HIV than for the HIV-negative population

100. The most frequently affected joint in acute gout is:
    a.   Knee
    b.   Ankle
    c.   Wrist
    d.   1st metatarsophalangeal joint
    e.   Midfoot

1. Answer a

Ig A nephropathy is the most common primary glomerulonephritis worldwide. It is an autoimmune condition characterised by IgA deposition in the renal mesangium on biopsy. 30-40% will develop a progressive renal disease. The disease burden is highest in East and South East Asia and this population also appears more likely to progress to advanced renal disease.[59,60]

2. Answer e

Löfgren syndrome is a presentation of sarcoidosis with erythema nodosum, arthritis, and bilateral hilar adenopathy on chest radiography. It is usually self-limiting with resolution in 3 to 6 months in most affected individuals. There may be associated fatigue and fever. Erythema nodosum is clinically and histologically indistinguishable from erythema nodosum from other causes. Histological confirmation is usually required for diagnosis of sarcoidosis but the presentation of erythema nodosum, arthritis, and bilateral hilar adenopathy on chest radiography is sufficient to diagnose Lofgren syndrome.[61]

3. Answer a

Heart failure with preserved ejection fraction (HFpEF) refers to heart failure with an ejection fraction of > 50%. Heart failure with reduced ejection fraction refers to heart failure with ejection fraction <40%. Heart failure with ejection fraction of 40-50% is referred to as heart failure with borderline preserved ejection fraction. The different entities have similar clinical presentations. HFrEF is more common than HFpEF. BNP can be useful in all types of heart failure, whether chronic or acute presentations.[56,57,58,67]

4. Answer b

Coronaviruses are single-stranded RNA viruses which can infect a large variety of animals as well as humans. Most strains of the virus cause self-limiting respiratory illnesses. New more pathogenic forms of the virus have emerged with SARS-CoV (severe acute respiratory syndrome coronavirus) in 2002 and MERS-CoV (Middle East respiratory syndrome coronavirus) in 2012. The SARS CoV epidemic originated in animal markets in south China and had a mortality of 10%. 80% of MERS cases occurred in Saudi Arabia with a mortality of 36%. Species jumping from animals to humans is believed to have been the origin of these strains. Coronaviruses may cause a variety of presentations from mild self-limiting respiratory infections to severe respiratory syndrome causing death. Lymphopenia is a common finding on laboratory analysis.[68]

SARS-CoV-2, a new strain of coronavirus which emerged from China in 2019 and caused the ongoing COVID-19 pandemic in 2020.

5. Answer d

1-2% of diabetes is a monogenic type known as maturity onset diabetes of the young (MODY). It is a distinct entity from type 1 and type 2 diabetes. The most common types involve genes encoding the enzyme glucokinase (GCK) and the nuclear transcription factors hepatocyte nuclear factor 1α (HNF1A) and hepatocyte nuclear factor 4α (HNF4A). HNF1A- MODY and HNF4A-MODY lead to progressively worsening hyperglycaemia into adulthood. They can lead to microvascular complications. They are not associated with insulin resistance but do not respond to insulin. Patients with these conditions are very sensitive to sulphonylureas which are usually the treatment of choice. Glucokinase (GCK) MODY causes long term stable hyperglycaemia which does not lead to microvascular complications and does not require treatment.[1]

6. Answer d

Bicuspid aortic valve is one of the most common congenital cardiac abnormalities and can lead to aortic valve and aortic root abnormalities as well as thoracic aortic aneurysm and dissection. Regular surveillance with transthoracic echocardiogram is required, usually every 5 to 10 years in those with no signs of aortic valve or ascending aorta abnormalities.[5]

7. Answer b

The START trial in 2015 showed the benefits in starting anti-retroviral treatment in HIV-positive individuals who are asymptomatic with high CD 4+ counts >500 cells per cubic millimetre. This also reduces an individual's risk of spreading the virus. AIDS can still occur even in those with good viral suppression. Poor compliance with treatment increases the risk of resistance and disease progression.[10]

8. Answer b

The most common complication of decompensated liver disease is ascites. Blood transfusion should be commenced in those with gastrointestinal bleeding and decompensated liver disease once Hb is less than 7 and aim for Hb of > 8 as more liberal transfusion policies may increase risk of rebleeding and death. Asterixis is diagnostic of hepatic encephalopathy, serum ammonia is not useful in acute assessment. A bowel frequency of 2 to 3 soft stools should be aimed for using lactulose to minimise bowel toxins. High volumes of 0.9% saline of 5% dextrose should be avoided as it may worsen ascites and 5% or 20% albumin is preferred for fluid replacement.[11]

9. Answer a

Marfan syndrome is an autosomal dominant condition characterised by mutations to the FBN 1 gene, affecting connective tissues. Diagnostic criteria focus on the presence of family history (not present in 25%), aortic root disease, ectopia lentis (lens dislocation, usually upward) and the presence of the FBN 1 gene. Although high-arched palate is a clinical feature it is not seen as been sufficiently discriminatory to be included in diagnostic criteria.[27,28]

10. Answer b

11. Answer c

Aortic stenosis is more common in the elderly and is most often due to valve calcification. In younger patients bicuspid aortic valve is the most common cause. Symptoms such as dyspnoea indicate more severe valve stenosis and herald the development of cardiac dysfunction. The prognosis is poor in untreated symptomatic aortic stenosis (50% survival at five years in those with angina). The outcome from surgical aortic valve replacement are generally good at all ages (89% survival at one year in octogenarians), with co-morbidity levels rather than age itself being a caution for surgery.[6]

12. Answer c

Adrenal crisis is a potentially life-threatening condition due to an absolute deficiency of cortisol. It may arise in the context of known or unknown adrenal insufficiency and can be primary or secondary. Autoimmune disease causes 80% of primary adrenal insufficiency (Addison's disease). Exogenous steroid use is one of the main causes of secondary adrenal insufficiency and stopping treatment abruptly may cause adrenal crisis.[73,74,75]

13. Answer e

Lung nodules are common radiological findings. Their management depends on clinical factors with smoking history and age being the most important. The most important imaging features of the nodule predicting malignancy are size (<6mm has <1% chance of being cancerous) and growth rate. The largest of multiple pulmonary nodules cannot be assumed to be the malignant one. Calcification, depending on the pattern, can be a predictor of a benign nodule. Fat attenuation can also be a predictor of a benign nodule.[76]

14. Answer c

PCR is the most common method for detecting respiratory viruses. Once collected the sample can be stored at room temperature for several days prior to testing. Storing in a fridge can reduce nucleic acid degradation. There is a high sensitivity (85-100%) and specificity (98-100%). It can detect live virus but also non-viable viruses so a test may remain positive even in the asymptomatic recovery period when a subject may not be infectious.[78]

15. Answer b

Aplastic anaemia is characterised by pancytopenia due to bone marrow failure and may be caused by

1. bone marrow damage, often iatrogenic, such as due to chemotherapy or radiation,

2. constitutional disorders which may be inherited, most commonly Fanconi anaemia

3. immune-mediated

Fanconi anaemia is an inherited disorder characterised by a variety of physical characteristics such as microcephaly, abnormal skin pigmentation and short stature, as well as pancytopenia and a precisposition to haematological and solid malignancy.[83,84]

Seckel syndrome is an inherited disorder characterised by microcephaly and intellectual disability, and some patients may develop pancytopenia.[83]

Dyskeratosis congenita is characterized by a classic triad of dysplastic nails, reticular pigmentation of the upper chest and/or neck, and oral leucoplakia. The classic triad may not be present in all individuals. Affected individuals are also at increased risk of aplastic anaemia, myelodysplastic syndrome and acute myelogenous leukaemia and some solid tumors.[86]

Diamond-Blackfan anaemia is characterized by a variable presentation which may include profound normochromic and usually macrocytic anaemia with normal leukocytes and platelets, congenital and growth retardation with a predisposition to acute myelogenous leukaemia, myelodysplastic syndrome and some solid tumours.[37]

Bloom syndrome is a rare inherited disorder characterised by short stature, microcephaly, intellectual disability and immunodeficiency as well as a predisposition to haematological and solid cancers.[85]

16. Answer e

Stevens-Johnson syndrome/toxic epidermal necrolysis (SJS/TEN) Is characterised by full thickness epidermal necrolysis. SJS/TEN exist on a spectrum, with Stevens-Johnson syndrome progressing to SJS/TEN overlap once >10% of body surface area has epidermal detachment, and SJS/TEN overlap progressing to TEN once > 30% of body surface area is involved. Systemic symptoms may precede mucosal symptoms by 1-3 days. Medication is a more common cause than infection, which is rare. The most important intervention is removing the causat ve agent as soon as possible. The evidence for corticosteroid use in SJS/TEN is conflicting.[92]

17. Answer e

Cross reactivity between penicillin and cephalosporin allergy occurs usually due to a reaction to the R1 side chain of the molecule rather than the central four-membered betalactam ring. Immediate or delayed hypersensitivity reactions may occur such as Stevens-Johnson syndrome and drug reaction with eosinophilia and systemic symptoms (DRESS) . True penicillin allergy is difficult to separate from a penicillin allergy label obtained after a childhood rash or other non severe adverse reactions, but it has been estimated that up to 90% of those with a label of penicillin allergy could safely take penicillins. Cross-reactivity with cephalosporins is less likely than previously described although is more likely to occur with first generation amino-cephalosporins such as cefalexin, with alternative cephalosporins likely to be safer. A label of penicillin allergy has been associated with an increased risk of adverse outcomes such as MRSA, clostridium difficile and vancomycin-resistant enterococci infection and colonisation.[95,96]

18. Answer d

The mechanisms of all the adverse effects of methotrexate are not completely understood. Some at least are related to its role as a folate antagonist and risk can be reduced with supplementation, such as cytopenias, stomatitis and nausea. There is evidence that folate supplementation may reduce the incidence of raised liver function blood tests, but liver fibrosis may be caused by other mechanisms. Pulmonary toxicity is thought to be an idiosyncratic reaction unrelated to folate deficiency. Skin nodulosis and renal toxicity are uncommon adverse effects of methotrexate, also unrelated to folate antagonism.[98]

19. Answer b

Primary ciliary dyskinesia (PCD) is an autosomal recessive disorder with heterogenous genotypes and phenotypes. It typically presents in early childhood with neonatal respiratory distress, oto-rhino-sinus disease and chronic productive cough. Most but not all men are infertile. Female subfertility occurs due to defects in fallopian tube ciliary function. There is also an increased risk of ectopic pregnancy. 50% have situs abnormalities such as situs inversus. Other clinical characteristics are pectus excavatum, asplenia and congenital heart disease.[99]

20. Answer a

Female gender confers an increased risk of stroke in the general population including those with atrial fibrillation. Obstructive sleep apnoea confers increased risk also although it is not included in risk stratification scores. . Heart failure confers increased risk whether reduced or preserved ejection fraction.[102]

21. Answer a

25 to 40% of non-Hodgkins lymphoma involves extranodal sites, with gastrointestinal the most common extranodal site, followed by the skin.[103]

22. Answer c

The malabsorption syndrome of diarrhoea, weight loss and asthenia is an uncommon presentation of coeliac disease in adults, with this presentation more common under three years of age Microcytic iron deficiency anaemia occurs in 40% of cases, more commonly than macrocytic anaemia due to B12 or folate deficiency. Raised liver transaminases will usually revert to normal 6 to 12 months after starting a gluten free diet. Thrombocytosis may be a marker for hyposplenism, as well as Howell Joly bodies in red cells on blood smear.[105]

23. Answer e

Acromegaly is caused by growth-hormone secreting somatotroph pituitary tumours. Sparsely granulated adenomas are more florid and aggressive. Growth hormone secretion is highly pulsatile and static testing is not useful for diagnosis. Elevated IGF1 (insulin-like growth factor 1) levels are specific but dynamic testing with a glucose tolerance test is required for diagnosis, showing a high nadir of growth hormone levels after a 75g glucose challenge. Treatment focusses on reducing mass effects of the tumour, and minimising cardiovascular, respiratory and metabolic effects. Surgical intervention may be required to control mass effects, and as 70% of tumours are invasive, they may not be fully resectable. Radiotherapy may cause long term side effects such as pituitary failure. Medical management includes treatment with dopamine agonists such as cabergoline which may control mild disease. Somatropin receptor ligands such as octreotide can control IGF1 and GH levels in 50-60%, with adenoma SST2 (somatostatin receptor subtype 2) expression, densely granulated adenoma and hypointensity on T2-weighted MRI markers of treatment responsiveness. 30% will get gastrointestinal side effects such as nausea and diarrhoea.

Intracranial pressure effects and sleep apnoea improve with successful treatment but hypertension may persist.[109]

24. Answer b

The Weber test is used to detect unilateral hearing loss and the sound is heard louder on the ipsilateral side in conductive hearing loss and the contralateral side in sensorineural hearing loss. It is useful in detecting a false negative Rinne test.[111]

25. Answer e

Thalidomide syndrome results from in-utero exposure to thalidomide. The most common feature is a shortened limb deformity known as phocomelia. Other features such as facial disfigurement, visual impairment, brain injury and internal organ derangement may also be features. The most common long term complication is musculoskeletal problems such as joint or muscle pains. This is at least partially attributable to an increased risk of osteoarthritis in the knees, hips and spine, but increased muscle tension and muscle weakness are also felt to contribute. Although the deformities of thalidomide syndrome are static the musculoskeletal pain worsens over time. Mental health problems such as depression are also prominent and related to severity of deformity.[113]

26. Answer e

Cushing disease refers specifically to excess adrenal cortisol production as a consequence of excess adrenocorticotropin hormone (ACTH) production from a pituitary adenoma. Cushing syndrome refers to a general state of hypercortisolism including exogenous steroids or an adrenal adenoma. Most Cushing syndrome arises from microadenomas <5mm and presentation with mass effects on local structures is uncommon. 40% are not apparent on imaging. Diagnosis is through dynamic testing such as a dexamethasone suppression test. Medical treatments are often unsatisfactory and transsphenoidal adenomectomy is the preferred treatment although recurrence may occur.[109,112]

27. Answer b

Chronic atrophic gastritis (CAG) is a chronic disease whose main features are atrophy or metaplasia of gastric glands. It may be autoimmune or associated with Helicobacter pylori infection. There may be distinguishing features between autoimmune and Helicobacter pylori-associated CAG (for example focal gastritis in H pylori associated and fundal and body involvement in autoimmune). In practice there is often considerable overlap even histologically. It presents insidiously and is usually quite advanced at the time of diagnosis. It may present with signs of iron or vitamin B12 deficiency, including anaemia. The neurological consequences of vitamin B12 deficiency may present, including neurological complications and depression. Diagnosis can be challenging. Serological tests such as anti-parietal cell antibodies may be non-specific, and it is best diagnosed by biopsy during endoscopy. CAG is a pre-malignant lesion with increased risk of intestinal type gastric cancer and gastric carcinoid.[115,116,117]

28. Answer d

Hidradenitis suppurativa is a chronic inflammatory skin condition characterised by painful subcutaneous nodules. About a third of those affected have a positive family history with an autosomal dominant pattern of inheritance. It is more common in women by a ratio of 3:1. It has been associated with a 'metabolic loop' of obesity, dyslipidaemia, hypertension and insulin resistance. Its pathogenesis and the role of bacteria remain uncertain, with multiple bacteria both aerobic and anaerobic isolated from lesions. Antibiotic treatment is used, with tetracyclines usually first line but other antibiotics also used such as clindamycin and rifampicin. It is uncertain if their efficacy in HS are due to antibacterial action or other factors such as anti-inflammatory or immunomodulatory activity. Biologic disease-modifying antirheumatic drugs (DMARDs) are used in treatment with adalimumab and infliximab showing good results in trials, and other agents being investigated.[119]

29. Answer e

Primary hyperparathyroidism most commonly arises due to a single parathyroid adenoma (80% of cases). Calcium levels may be normal (normocalcaemic hyperparathyroidism) when renal stones are less likely but the bone complications such as osteoporosis and increased fracture risk may still occur. Vitamin D deficiency can worsen hyperparathyroidism and vitamin D supplements should be given if appropriate. Surgery is the definitive treatment but is not always needed. Current indications for surgery include particularly high calcium levels, age less than 50 years, osteoporosis or fragility fracture history, renal impairment, renal stones and high urinary calcium levels. Parathyroid imaging such as ultrasound, MRI or sestamibi scan are needed only for localisation prior to surgery and not for diagnosis.[122]

30. Answer c

Betablockers such as atenolol are Vaughan Williams Class II anti-arrhythmics. Class I anti-arrhythmics are sodium channel blockers, with subdivisions depending on effect on repolarisation and 'refractoriness'. Class III are potassium channel blockers such as amiodarone. Class IV are calcium channel blockers.[124]

31. Answer d

Bechet's disease is a chronic inflammatory vasculitis affecting multiple organ systems with features of both an autoimmune and autoinflammatory condition. There is a clustering along the ancient Silk Road between Asia and Southern Europe. Oral, genital and skin manifestations are common and recurrent oral ulceration is a requisite for diagnosis under current International Classification Criteria of Bechet's. Although there may be some small overlap with joint involvement and spondyloarthropathies, there is not a HLA B27 association as such. The most common genetic association is with HLA B51 but this accounts for less then 20% of genetic risk, so other unknown genetic factors are suspected. Blood testing is not useful for diagnosis with often normal inflammatory markers and no useful serological tests. Ocular involvement is common and sight threatening. Renal involvement is rare.[126]

32. Answer a

The most common genetic mutation in haemochromatosis is a G-to-A missense mutation leading to the substitution of tyrosine for cysteine at amino acid position 282 of the protein product (C282Y). It is an autosomal recessive condition so only homozygotes usually manifest the disease, with variable penetrance. C282Y homozygotes constitute 80% of those with haemochromatosis. Heterozygotes are carriers. The other two identified mutations associated with haemochromatosis are H63D and S65C.[128]

33. Answer e

Epworth sleepiness scale is a questionnaire scale used to assess excessive daytime sleepiness. It rates 0-3 for sleepiness in eight situations during an individual's day. A score of less than 10 is considered normal, with a score greater than 16 considered severe excessive daytime sleepiness. It is not sensitive or specific for obstructive sleep apnoea diagnosis. It may be subject to secondary gain when used in screening, for example in commercial drivers who may underreport symptoms in case it may affect ability to work.[132,133]

34. Answer a

Hyperthyroidism reduces total cholesterol levels which will rise once euthyroidism is established. Hypothyroidism is associated with a rise in LDL levels. Overt hyperthyroidism is associated with increased cardiovascular morbidity and mortality, mainly due to the increased risk of heart failure and atrial fibrillation. It also increases stroke risk due to the increased risk of atrial fibrillation. Atrial fibrillation is found in 10-15% of those with hyperthyroidism as compared with 0.5% of the general population. Subclinical hyperthyroidism occurs when TSH is low with normal thyroid hormone levels, and is also associated with increased cardiovascular risk through increased risk of atrial fibrillation and heart failure. Consideration should be given to treating subclinical hyperthyroidism particularly in those with a very suppressed TSH and over 65 years or age or with cormorbidities.[134]

35. Answer d

D Dimer is a biomarker of fibrin activity and degradation and serves as an indirect marker of thrombotic activity. It has been mostly used in the exclusion of venous thromboembolic disease to try and avoid costly radiological testing. It has been studied in several other contexts, with conflicting results. It has been shown to be of use in predicting thromboembolic risk in hospitalised medically ill patients at increased risk of thromboembolic disease who may benefit from extended courses of thromboprophylaxis. When high sensitivity tests are used it is useful in excluding venous thromboembolic disease, disseminated intravascular coagulation and aortic dissection but given its low specificity a positive test is insufficient for diagnosing these conditions. It has been shown to be not useful in predicting stroke risk in atrial fibrillation, predicting cardiovascular risk in those with HIV or the general population and in identifying acute coronary syndrome in those with chest pain.[135]

36. Answer d

Ebola virus disease is caused by Ebola virus species causing periodic outbreaks in humans in Africa since 1976. It begins with a non-specific viral illness progressing within a few days to gastrointestinal symptoms and potential profound fluid loss of up to 10 litres per day. Haemorrhagic complications occur in less than half of those affected. The most common method of diagnosis is quantitative real time polymerase chain reaction (qRT-PCR). Promising treatments have been developed and include the monoclonal-antibody cocktails ZMapp and REGN-EB3, a single monoclonal antibody MAb114, and remdesivir, a small-molecule antiviral drug. Vaccines have also been developed, with the most promising at present a single-shot, live-attenuated vaccine based on a recombinant vesicular stomatitis virus expressing the Zaire ebolavirus glycoprotein. This vaccine showed excellent results when tested in the West African outbreak from 2013-2016. The mainstay of outbreak management remains identifying and isolating cases. Contacts of cases need to be followed up for 21 days, the maximum incubation period.[138]

37. Answer d

Breast feeding, previous appendicectomy and active smoking all reduce risk of developing ulcerative colitis (UC) and there is no gender difference in incidence. Use of non-steroidal anti-inflammatory medications and hormonal contraception and replacement therapy are associated with increased risk but not antibiotic use.[142]

38. Answer e

The Modified Duke Criteria use major and minor criteria for diagnosis of infective endocarditis. Major criteria include blood culture positivity for a typical microorganism (for example viridans group streptococci, staphylococcus aureus among others) or persistent bacteraemia, positive serology for coxiella burnetii and echocardiographic findings typical of valve vegetation, abscess or new dehiscence of prosthetic valve or new valvular regurgitation. Minor criteria include predisposing conditions of intravenous drug use or a predisposing cardiac condition, as well as vascular phenomena such as arterial embolism, septic pulmonary emboli, mycotic aneurysm, intracranial haemorrhage, conjunctival haemorrhages or Janeway's lesions. The diagnosis can be classified as definite, possible or rejected. Definite infective endocarditis requires two major criteria, one major and three minor or five minor.[143,144]

39. Answer c

Metformin associated lactic acidosis (MALA) is a rare event with an estimated incidence of 0.03 to 0.06 per 1000 patient years. It tends to occur in those with underlying pre-existing conditions such as renal impairment in combination with an acute exacerbating event such as dehydration or sepsis. It may occur in those with mild renal dysfunction or on usual doses of metformin. It has a high fatality rate of 30-50%. Biguanides were developed in the 1950s to treat type 2 diabetes. Phenformin is the biguanide most likely to cause lactic acidosis, 20 times more likely than metformin. Early experiences with phenformin led to caution at the introduction of metformin and advice against its use in renal or hepatic insufficiency, heart failure and the very elderly. The emergence of metformin as a first line agent in the treatment of type 2 diabetes has led to concerns that these guidelines may be too conservative given the rare incidence of MALA. However there is also a belief that the rare occurrence may be due to these conservative guidelines. The guidelines regarding use of metformin in at-risk conditions varies between different jurisdictions.[147]

40. Answer a

α - thalassaemia is a haemoglobinopathy arising die to defects in the α haemoglobin chain. More than 100 generic forms have been identified, and the severity usually correlates with the number of non-functioning gene copies. Severe forms can lead to hydrops fetalis or require regular transfusions. Milder forms may have low mean corpuscular volume and mean corpuscular haemoglobin with normal or mildly low haemoglobin and needs to be distinguished from iron deficiency.[146]

41. Answer c

Aspirin is the most effective antiplatelet agent for reducing risk of stroke recurrence after an initial noncardioembolic event, and the addition of clopidogrel has been associated with increased benefit in the first 21 days.[150]

42. Answer e

The negative predictive value of a test refers to post-test probability that a person with a negative test result does not have the condition. It can be calculated as:

true negatives / (false negatives + true negatives)

The post-test probability that a person with a positive test result has the condition is the positive predictive value.

The proportion of people without a condition who have a negative test result is the specificity of a test.

The proportion of people with a condition with a given test result (either positive or negative) divided by the proportion of people without the condition with that result is the likelihood ratio.[151]

43. Answer d

Tumour lysis syndrome (TLS) is a biochemical complication of rapid cell breakdown associated with malignancy. It usually arises as a result of chemotherapy for haematological malignancies such as lymphoma, leukaemia or multiple myeloma. The biochemical abnormalities which occur in TLS are hyperkalaemia, hyperphosphataemia, hyperuricaemia and hypocalcaemia.[152]

44. Answer a

Membranous nephropathy (MN) is the most common cause of nephrotic syndrome in white adults. It usually presents with severe proteinuria, oedema, hypoalbuminaemia and hyperlipidaemia. Most cases are primary MN, with about 20% of cases secondary to other conditions, such as autoimmune conditions (SLE, rheumatoid arthritis), infection (hepatitis B and C) malignancy (colon or lung cancer) and drugs (gold, penicillamine). It is more likely to be secondary in children than in adults. In patients older than 60 years of age, MN is associated with malignancy in 20-30% of cases. Spontaneous remission occurs in 30% but 30-40% will progress to end stage renal failure within 5 to 15 years. Conservative treatment involves statin use, thromboprophylaxis and angiotensin II blockade with ACE inhibitors or angiotensin II receptor blockers. However the decrease in proteinuria is unlikely to exceed 30% compared with pretreatment values so will not eliminate proteinuria in those with nephrotic syndrome and heavy proteinuria. Primary membranous nephropathy is associated with antibodies against specific podocyte antigens, in particular M-type phospholipase A2 receptor (PLA$_2$R). These antibodies can be found in the blood and on staining renal biopsies, and the level found can be correlated with chances of spontaneous remission, response to immunosuppression, time to remission, relapse risk and progression to nephrotic syndrome and progressive renal failure.[154,155]

45. Answer b

Hypersensitivity pneumonitis is a delayed allergic reaction to external agents leading to inflammation of the alveoli, terminal bronchioles and alveolar interstitium. Diagnosis can be difficult as a gold standard test is not available. Diagnosis depends on the presence of typical clinical features, radiology and lung function testing and possibly identification of precipitins to a known causative agent. However not all causative agents can be identified on serological testing, and may be present in those exposed without hypersensitivity pneumonitis. In 2003 a HP working group identified six predictive criteria in diagnosis: (1) exposure to a known causative antigen, (2) presence of precipitins to the suspected causative antigen, (3) recurrent respiratory and systemic symptoms, (4) inspiratory crackles detected by physical examination, (5) symptoms occurring 4–8 hours after exposure, (6) weight loss.[156,157]

46. Answer d

Wilson's disease may be characterised by a variety of psychiatric presentations, occurring at any age and have been described even in the very young. Wilson's disease itself is notable for its variation of presentations whether neurological or hepatic. Psychosis, personality disorder, behavioural disorder, attention deficit hyperactivity disorder, catatonia and eating disorders have all been described, but the most common manifestation is mood disorder.[208]

47. Answer c

Psoriasis is a chronic inflammatory condition with plaques involving the entire thickness of the skin. 40% of those affected will develop psoriatic

arthropathy. Nail involvement occurs in over half of those affected with psoriasis and up to 80% of those with psoriatic arthropathy. 15% may have nail involvement only.[158]

48. Answer d

Bisphosphonates are stable analogues of pyrophosphate compounds and are the most widely prescribed treatments for osteoporosis at present. They reduce the risk of vertebral fracture by 40-70% and hip fractures by 40-50%.[160]

49. Answer a

There are several risk factors associated with type 1 diabetes development including dietary and lifestyle factors, vitamin D sufficiency, early life exposure to viruses and decreased gut-microbiome diversity. Although usually associated with type 2 diabetes, obesity is a risk factor for type 1 diabetes development also with β cell stress a possible mechanism. Most individuals with type 1 diabetes do not achieve recommended Hb A1c targets. Diabetic ketoacidosis causes a larger proportion of type 1 diabetes related deaths (13-19%) than hypoglycaemic events (4-10%). Microvascular complications manifest mainly as retinopathy, neuropathy or nephropathy but can also affect cognitive function, the heart and other organs. Macrovascular complications are the major cause of premature morbidity and mortality.[161]

50. Answer a

Factors associated with disease progression to cirrhosis include male gender, developing hepatitis C infection when older than 40 years of age, HIV or HBV coinfection, alcohol consumption of at least 50 g per day and immunosuppression.[162,163]

51. Answer a

Symmetrical arthritis is not included in the diagnostic criteria for rheumatoid arthritis (RA) to allow for early asymmetric presentation of RA.[164,165]

The 2010 American College of Rheumatology/European League Against Rheumatism classification criteria for diagnosis of RA are:

A	Joint involvement	
	One large joint	0
	Two to 10 large joints	1
	One to three small joints	2
	Four to ten small joints	3
	>10 joints (at least one small joint)	5
B	Serology	
	Negative RF and ACPA	0
	Low positive RF or low positive ACPA	2
	High positive RF or high positive ACPA	3
C	Acute phase reactant	
	Normal CRP and ESR	0
	Abnormal CRP or abnormal ESR	1
D	Duration of symptoms	
	< 6 weeks	0
	6 weeks or more	1

52. Answer a

The most commonly documented drug allergy in medical records is to penicillin.[166]

53. Answer b

Thyroid dysfunction is a common side effect of lithium treatment. It most commonly presents as subclinical hypothyroidism, and may present as overt hypothyroidism or goitre. Symptoms are similar to hypothyroidism in other forms of hypothyroidism and can be similar to depression, so clinical features are insufficient for diagnosis and thyroid function tests are required for diagnosis. The risk is higher by a factor of 8 in those with antithyroid antibodies, with female gender, older age and a family history of hypothyroidism other risk factors. Lithium treatment does not need to be stopped and hypothyroidism can be treated in the usual with way with thyroxine replacement.[169]

54. Answer d

Subacute combined immunodeficiency (SCID) is a genetic disorder characterised by reduced T lymphocytes and variable amounts of B lymphocytes. It is uniformly fatal in newborns if not diagnosed early and treated. It presents with repeated severe infections in infancy. Early treatment with enzyme treatment or haemopoietic stem cell transplantation reduces mortality. SCID be screened for with an assay to detect T cell receptor excision circle which is done on a Guthrie card, and neonatal screening is now routine in many jurisdictions.[171,172]

55. Answer a

Congenital heart disease occurs in 44% of those with Down syndrome, with ASD the most common comprising 45% and VSD comprising 35%.[175]

56. Answer e

Transfusion-associated circulatory overload (TACO) is defined as acute pulmonary oedema within 6 hours of transfusion with evidence of circulatory overload (three or more of acute respiratory distress, radiographic pulmonary oedema, elevated central venous pressure, evidence of left heart failure, elevated BNP, positive fluid balance). The primary mitigation strategies are slowing of transfusion rates and prophylactic volume reduction with diuretics.

Transfusion-related acute lung injury (TRALI) is another potentially fatal blood transfusion reaction and is defined as onset of acute pulmonary oedema within 6 hours of completion of blood product transfusion without circulatory overload or acute respiratory distress syndrome (ARDS) risk factors. It is antibody mediated and mitigation strategies are use of male-only blood product sources (risk is increased in products from previously pregnant women due to alloimmunisation), screening donors for antibodies and through pooling blood products from many donors, which dilutes any antibodies present.[176]

57. Answer a

Trousseau's signs is carpopedal spasm after inflation of a sphygmomanometer above the systolic blood pressure and is seen in hypocalcaemia.[177]

58. Answer b

Up to 30% of acute lower motor neurone facial palsy may have a cause other than Bells palsy. Acute suppurative ear disease, Ramsay Hunt syndrome, parotid tumour and Lyme disease are potential differentials. Upper facial muscle sparing suggests an upper motor neurone weakness and an alternative diagnosis.[178]

59. Answer e

Water deprivation test is useful to distinguish between central diabetes insipidus, nephrogenic diabetes insipidus and primary polydipsia. Diabetes insipidus is an abnormality of vasopressin production or function. Central diabetes insipidus occurs due to a problem with vasopressin at the pituitary gland and nephrogenic diabetes insipidus occurs due to abnormal action of vasopressin at the kidneys. A water deprivation test involves depriving the patient of water and assessing the response. It is potentially dangerous and should be performed by specialists in the hospita setting with continued measurement of serum and urine osmolality, urine volume and weight. If urine output falls and urine osmolality exceeds 750mOsm/kg then diabetes insipidus is excluded. Desmopressin is then given in those with confirmed diabetes insipidus, and those with nephrogenic diabetes insipidus will not respond.[209]

60. Answer d

Sticky platelet syndrome is an autosomal dominant familial disorder of platelet hypercoagulability. It is associated with increased risk of arterial and venous thrombosis as well as migraine with aura and pregnancy complications. There may be atypical thrombosis sites such as cerebral sinuses or retina.[180]

61. Answer d

Porphyrias consist of nine conditions characterised by alterations in enzymes involved in heme biosynthesis. There is overproduction of heme precursors in either the liver or bone marrow, leading to a classification of porphyrias as either hepatic or erythropoietic. Porphyria cutanea tarda is the most common form of porphyria. It is a hepatic porphyria which manifests as blistering photosensitive skin rash with bullae and skin fragility usually on the backs of the hands. It does not have neurological manifestations. It is the only porphyria that can develop without an inherited mutation of an affected gene. Only 20% of those with PCT have a heterozygous uroporphyrinogen decarboxylase (UROD) mutation with other factors required for clinical manifestation of the disease. These factors include alcohol, smoking, hepatitis C, HIV, oestrogen in females, hemochromatosis mutations as well as UROD mutations. It is an iron related disorder, with an association with liver iron overload, and phlebotomy is an effective treatment. Iron deficiency is protective and the disease can worsen with iron supplements. Low dose hydroxychloroquine is also an effective treatment.[181]

62. Answer a

Paget's disease of bone is a disorder of bone turnover, characterised by abnormalities in osteoclast and osteoblast function leading to foci of disordered bone formation. Its cause is unknown, with genetic predisposition combining with unknown environmental triggers to cause foci of abnormal bone formation. Axial skeleton lesions are prominent but any bone can be affected. Lesions are not inflammatory or neoplastic. Plain x rays are usually sufficient for diagnosis, with a typical appearance of clearly demarcated Pagetic lesions with evidence of osteolysis, coarsening of trabecular pattern, sclerosis and bone deformity. Radionuclide scans show lesions but appearances are less specific, but they are useful for assessing extent of disease. Affected sites will not migrate to other bones spontaneously but transference to another bone has been describes after bone grafting.

A single treatment with a potent bisphosphonate has been shown to stop disease in up to 90% of cases.[182,183]

63. Answer e

Rabies is a viral infection caused by a virus of the rhabdoviridae family of viruses. It is usually transmitted via a bite or scratch from any infected mammal, via saliva. The five stages are incubation, prodrome, acute neurologic illness, coma and death. Incubation may take days to years. The virus causes a neuroencephalitis, with an encephalitic category ('furious') and paralytic category ('dumb'). The encephalitic form presents in 85% of cases and the paralytic form is less common occurring in about 20%. Early wound treatment is essential and can be life-saving. In the unvaccinated, early treatment with vaccination on days 0,3,7 and 14 and rabies immunoglobulin is essential, and should be initiated for any situation where rabies is even a remote possibility. The vaccinated should also have early vaccination at days 0 and 3. Once symptoms develop death is inevitable.[184,185,186]

64. Answer a

Bedbugs are Cimex lectularis (common bedbug) and Cimex hemipterus (tropical bed bugs).[187]

65. Answer a

Atrial fibrillation secondary to hyperthyroidism is more likely to cause stroke than atrial fibrillation without associated hyperthyroidism.

Hyperthyroidism is a state of increased production and secretion of thyroid hormone from the thyroid gland. Radioactive iodine uptake by the thyroid gland is increased in true hyperthyroidism.

Thyrotoxicosis is a clinical syndrome of excess circulating thyroid hormone of any cause. Exogenous thyroid hormone is a cause of thyrotoxicosis and radioactive iodine uptake by the thyroid gland is not increased in those with thyrotoxicosis from exogenous sources.

The treatments for hyperthyroidism are antithyroid drugs, radioiodine or thyroidectomy. All three are suitable in Graves' disease, but antithyroid drugs should not be used in toxic adenoma or toxic multinodular goitre as these patients rarely go into remission.

Propylthiouracil is the preferred antithyroid medication in pregnancy, and thiamazone may be used after the first trimester.[188]

66. Answer a

Kimmelstiel-Wilson nodules are renal nodular lesions consisting of areas of marked mesangial expansion forming large round fibrillar mesangial zones and are seen in diabetic glomerulosclerosis.[189,190,191]

67. Answer d

Respiratory failure occurs due to a failure of ventilation (movement of gas in and out of the lungs) or gas exchange (transferring oxygen from air to blood and transferring carbon dioxide from blood to air).

Type 1 respiratory failure occurs when there is hypoxia with normal or low carbon dioxide in the blood (<6kPa). It represents a failure of gas exchange, with the increased solubility of carbon dioxide in the blood preventing hypercapnia.

Type 2 respiratory failure occurs when there is hypoxia with high carbon dioxide in the blood (>6kPa). It represents a failure of lung ventilation with or without failure of gas exchange.

Hypoventilation may occur due to neuromuscular disease, opiate toxicity, reduced chest wall compliance in obesity and iatrogenic over-oxygenation (reduced hypoxic drive).

Severe COVID-19 pneumonia is more likely to cause type 1 respiratory failure due to severe acute respiratory distress syndrome and its effects on gas exchange. Hence the level of hypoxia may seem out of proportion to the level of respiratory distress, as gas exchange is affected more than ventilation. Type 2 respiratory failure may occur in those prone to hypoventilation (for example COPD) or with very severe disease and fatigue.[214]

68. Answer c

Primary aldosteronism (Conn's syndrome) is the most common cause of secondary hypertension and is estimated to cause 8-10% of cases of hypertension. It is estimated to cause 20% of cases of refractory hypertension.[192,193]

69. Answer a

Dexamethasone was shown to reduce mortality in this with severe COVID 19 requiring ventilatory support and supplemental oxygen.[194]

In preliminary reports remdesivir was shown to shorten time to recovery in COVID 19 but improvements in mortality did not reach statistical significance.[195]

Early reports on hydroxychloroquine use have not shown benefit in COVID 19.

An early study with a lopinavir-ritonavir combination did not show benefit in COVID 19.[196]

70. Answer b

Intervertebral disks are essentially avascular and depend on diffusion of nutrients and waste through the capillary bed of the adjacent vertebral end plates. End plate calcification can affect disk homeostasis, leading to the death of intervertebral disk cells. This leads to fissuring of the annulus fibrosis on the exterior border of the disk, resulting in the herniation of the central nucleus pulposus. This results in the transfer of load sharing from the nucleus pulposus to the annulus fibrosis. Nociceptive pain fibres in the annulus fibrosis and nucleus pulposis become sensitised by the inflammatory environment, although neck pain may also occur from adjacent soft tissues and facet joints and possibly from central nervous system sensitisation.[198]

71. Answer d

Chronic lymphocytic leukaemia is a malignancy of CD5+ lymphocytes characterised by accumulation of small, mature-appearing lymphocytes in the blood, bone marrow and secondary lymphoid tissues. It can be divided into two main subsets depending on whether cels express a mutated or unmutated immunoglobulin heavy-chain variable region gene (IGHV).

Unmutated IGHV expression reflects a pre-germinal centre origin for the affected IGHV expression reflects a pre-germinal centre origin for the affected malignant cells and is associated with more aggressive disease. Mutated IGHV reflects post germinal centre cell origin. The geminal centres are sites in the lymph nodes where B cells undergo somatic hypermutation in their immunoglobulin variable region genes during immune process selection, which is a normal course of events. 80% of those with CLL carry at least one of four chromosomal alterations: del(13q), del(11q), del(17p) and trisomy 12.

Del (13q) is the most common affecting over 50% of those with CLL and is associated with a favourable prognosis.

Transmission of CLL via blood transfusion has not been described.

It is the most common adult leukaemia in western countries but is much less common in Asia. Incidence increases with increasing age.[199,200]

72. Answer c

Lung cancer staging is essential for determining appropriate treatment in both small cell and non-small cell lung cancer. Surgical resection is potentially curative in stages IA, IB, IIA and IIB non-small cell lung cancer. Staging is useful in small cell lung cancer to determine if radiotherapy is indicated for localised disease.

The TNM staging system is used with T denoting primary tumour size (for example T1 indicates tumour up to 3cm, T2 tumour 3-5cm etc), N denoting sites of nodal involvement and M denoting other sites of more distant metastases. The International Association for the Study of Lung Cancer revised system of classification for lung cancer stages from 0 to IVB depending on extent of disease. Stage 0 includes carcinoma in situ (TisN0M0).

CT scan is the most widely used modality for lung cancer staging, but is limited in differentiating benign from malignant nodules. FDG PET scanning has shown increased sensitivity but is expensive and less widely available.[201,202,203]

73. Answer a

Pulmonary hypertension is a severe vascular disorder defined as mean pulmonary arterial pressure of 25mmHg or more at rest. It is subdivided into 5 groups depending on cause. Pulmonary arterial hypertension describes a subgroup with pulmonary arterial pressure of 25mmHg or greater as well as normal pulmonary capillary wedge pressure of 15mmHg or less and pulmonary vascular resistance of greater than 3 Wood units, and where other common causes of pulmonary hypertension such as chronic lung disease, chronic pulmonary thromboembolic disease or left heart failure are not present.

Oxygen is only indicated in the presence of hypoxaemia. Anticoagulation is only indicated if there is a specific indication such as chronic

thromboembolic pulmonary disease. Diuresis is only required if there are signs of volume overload. Maintaining fitness and exercise should be encouraged unless there are other specific contraindications.

Calcium channel blockers are indicated in a subgroup of patients with pulmonary arterial hypertension, where a vasoreactivity test during cardiac catheterisation demonstrates a fall in mean pulmonary arterial pressure of more than 10mmHg to less than 40mmHg without a drop in cardiac output.[204,205]

74. Answer d

Epistaxis is the most common site of bleeding in hereditary haemorrhagic telangiectasia occurring in 96% of those with the condition.[204]

75. Answer a

There is a history of asbestos exposure in about 80% of cases of mesothelioma. There is a long latency period of 15-50 years with a median of about 40 years. It is most commonly associated with exposure to amphibole asbestos fibres. There is an inconsistent link with Simian virus 40. 70-80% of mesotheliomas arise from the pleura with the remainder mostly involving the peritoneum. Pericardial mesothelioma is rare.[206]

76. Answer d

Kayser-Fleischer rings occur in Wilson's disease due to accumulation of copper in the Descement membrane. They can be seen as brown, golden or green colouration at the periphery of the cornea. They require slit lamp examination for proper diagnosis. Similar changes may be seen in neoplastic conditions with high serum copper such as multiple myeloma, and in primary biliary cirrhosis and cholestasis. They are present in 100% of those with neurological Wilson's disease, 50% of those with hepatic disease and 30% of those with presymptomatic disease.[208]

77. Answer c

Diabetes insipidus is a rare condition caused by an abnormality of vasopressin function. It may be due to problems with vasopressin production in the pituitary gland (central diabetes insipidus) or the effect of vasopressin on the kidneys (nephrogenic diabetes insipidus). It is characterised by severe thirst and polyuria. If 24 hour urinary volume is less than 2.5 litres then diabetes insipidus is unlikely.[209]

78. Answer d

Anosmia is loss of sense of smell and may be conductive (physical barriers preventing odorants reaching the olfactory system) or central (problems with the olfactory system detecting odorants).

It occurs in around one half of patients with COVID-19 and may be associated with loss of taste. It resolves in 90% of these patients within four weeks. There can be associated loss of taste, although whether this is due to an independent gustatory dysfunction is uncertain. When caused by COVID-19 it is usually accompanied by other symptoms but may be an isolated symptom in 10%. Oral corticosteroids have not been shown to help.[211]

79. Answer d

Faecal microbiota transplantation (FMT) involves replacing the normal gut microbiota and is a promising treatment for clostridioides difficile infection (CDI). Antibiotic therapy can significantly reduce the amount of intestinal microbiota and it is thought that Bacteroides and Firmicutes in particular play an immunological role in the defence against CDI. Studies have shown FMT have curative rates of 81% versus 31% in vancomycin alone treatment. FMT can be given via oral capsule, retention enema or colonoscopy. The procedures have not yet been standardised. Donated samples may be frozen and used within 5 to 6 months. Potential donors need to be screened for viral, bacterial and parasitic infection.[244]

80. Answer e

Bacillus Calmette-Guerin (BCG) vaccination is a live attenuated form of Mycobacterium bovis. It is used to protect against tuberculosis. It is a live vaccine and should not be given to the immunosuppressed. It is known to be efficacious in preventing disseminated infection in children but its efficacy is much less certain in adults. Disseminated BCG infection has been described after vaccination in the immunosuppressed, and after bladder cancer treatment, which may not emerge for many years. Whether it is given to newborns or healthcare workers depends largely on the prevalence in the community and individual risk.

It is administered intravesically in the treatment of superficial bladder cancer.[215,216,217]

81. Answer b

Rheumatic heart disease is the most common predisposing factor for native valve endocarditis in developing countries less common that the other factors listed in developed nations.[218]

82. Answer b

2015 EULAR-ACR recommendations for initial treatment of polymyalgia rheumatica is oral prednisolone 12.5mg-25mg per day. Higher doses are recommended if there are risks of relapse or prolonged therapy and lower doses if there are risk factors for adverse reactions to oral corticosteroids.[219,220,221]

83. Answer d

Postural tachycardia syndrome (POTS) is a syndrome characterised by chronic symptoms of orthostatic intolerance with sustained and excessive sinus tachycardia in the absence of orthostatic hypotension. Diagnosis depends on the chronicity of symptoms and the demonstration of a sustained increase in heart rate of 30 bpm or more within 10 minutes of standing in the absence of a postural drop in blood pressure. Frequent associations include female gender, joint hypermobility, chronic fatigue syndrome, fibromyalgia, migraine, bowel irregularities and autoimmune disorders Symptoms of orthostatic intolerance include lightheadedness, palpitations, chest pain or discomfort, dyspnoea and syncope. Peripheral acrocyanosis may also occur, which is a red-blue discoloration of the legs that is cold to touch. Other causes such as hyperthyroidism or cardiac dysrhythmia must be excluded and ablation is not useful without an associated dysrhythmia.[222]

84. Answer a

Ehlers Danlos syndrome (EDS) is a heterogenous group of monogenic disorders characterised by generalised connective tissue fragility. Clinical features include skin hyperextensibility and fragility, vascular fragility and easy bruising, variable bleeding tendency and joint hypermobility. Rapid gene sequencing has led to several subtypes being identified, with clinical manifestations varying from asymptomatic to potentially life threatening. Most of the EDS subtypes are caused by defects in fibrillary collagen types I, III and V. Hypermobile EDS has considerable clinical overlap with joint hypermobility syndrome and as no genetic cause has been identified for either, some believe them to be interchangeable terms. The Brighton criteria are used to diagnose joint hypermobility syndrome and the Villefranche criteria to diagnose EDS.[223]

85. Answer b

Trigeminal neuralgia is characterised by severe short spasms of pain occurring in the distribution of one or more branches of the trigeminal nerve.

Trigeminal neuralgia may be classical, secondary or idiopathic. Classical is the most common and is caused by intracranial vascular compression of the trigeminal nerve root. Secondary trigeminal neuralgia occurs in 15% of cases and is due to an underlying neurological cause such as multiple sclerosis or a benign cerebellopontine angle tumour. Idiopathic causes account for about 10% of cases. [224]

86. Answer e

Post-acute COVID-19 symptoms (or long COVID-19) are symptoms lasting more than three weeks in those with a previous diagnosis of COVID-19, and the array of symptoms at the time of writing is enormous. Given the variation in testing availability of COVID-19 at the time of writing, as well as the uncertainly around false negative rates, it is suggested that a positive COVID-19 test should not be a prerequisite for diagnosis. It appears to be relatively common in those who have had mild symptoms. Around 10% of those with COVID-19 remain unwell after three weeks although higher rates are quoted in some studies. The most common symptoms are cough, low grade fever and fatigue, but many symptoms are described. The challenge facing physicians is identifying mild symptoms likely to resolve from those indicating a serious post-COVID-19 diagnosis such as pericarditis or pulmonary embolus. Psychological features such as anxiety and low mood can also be a feature.[225]

87. Answer c

Colour vision deficiency is one of the most common visual problems and can be divided into acquired or congenital. Congenital colour vision deficiency is usually X-linked and most commonly affects red-green colour vision. Ishihara's test was developed in 1906 and is still the most widely used test for detecting colour vision deficiency. It is used mainly as a screening test for detecting red-green colour vision deficiency and does not have tritan (blue) plates. It has been shown to be highly sensitive and specific for red-green colour deficiency screening purposes (both 0.85 to 0.95). It has limitations and cannot provide information on the severity of colour vision deficiency. It is available in 24 and 38-plate editions.[226,227]

88. Answer d

Thyroid nodules are common and often detected incidentally on radiology performed for another reason. All patients with an incidentally detected thyroid nodule should have a dedicated ultrasound to assess the thyroid gland and neck. Features suggestive of a malignant nodule are microcalcifications, hypoechogenicity of the nodule compared with the surrounding gland parenchyma, irregular margins and shape taller than wide on transverse view. Hyperfunctioning nodules are less likely to be malignant than non-functioning nodules. Fine needle aspirate is preferred to core needle biopsy to obtain a tissue diagnosis due to higher risk of bleeding with core needle biopsy.

Management of thyroid nodules depends on risk of malignancy based on ultrasound features and thyroid cytopathology based on the Bethesda criteria. Nodules >4cm diameter should be considered for surgical intervention even with benign cytology as there is a higher risk of sampling error and a higher risk of false negatives with larger nodules.[228,229]

89. Answer c

Primary biliary cirrhosis is an autoimmune disorder of the liver characterised by chronic biochemical cholestasis, positive anti-mitochondrial antibodies and liver histology showing nonsuppurative destructive cholangitis and interlobular bile duct destruction.

Anti-mitochondrial antibodies (AMA) are detected in >90% of those with primary biliary cirrhosis. AMAs are detected in <1% of the general population and in 8% of those with hepatitis C infection.

Of those in the general population with positive anti-mitochondrial antibodies without primary biliary cirrhosis, 10% will subsequently develop the condition. In those in the general population with positive anti-mitochondrial antibodies without primary biliary cirrhosis annual liver blood monitoring is recommended.[231]

90. Answer b

QT interval was not seen as a significant source of pathology when ECG waveforms were described first in the late 19th century. The discovery of this family in 1957 led to the realisation of the potential for aberrant QT intervals to be a pathological entity and to cause sudden death.

Congenital long QT syndromes are characterised by syncopal episodes and sudden death. All associated genes encode cardiac ion channel subunits or proteins involved in modulating ionic currents.

Jervell Lange Nielson syndrome is congenital long QT syndrome associated with congenital deafness. It is autosomal recessive occurring due to mutations in either the KCNQ1 or KCNE1 genes. It is one of the more severe forms of congenital long QT syndrome with 90% of those affected having cardiac events, and 50% affected by the age of 3 years. The usual treatments for congenital long QT syndrome such as betablockers and left cardiac sympathetic denervation may be less effective in this syndrome and implantable cardioverter defibrillator should be seriously considered.[232,233]

91. Answer e

Gabapentinoids are anticonvulsant medications that have been repurposed as analgesic and anxiety medications. Pregabalin is 6 times more potent in its receptor binding than gabapentin and is absorbed more quickly, reaching maximum plasma concentrations in one hour as opposed to 3 to 4 hours for gabapentin. The bioavailability of pregabalin remains at 90% even at very high dosages but bioavailability is only 60% for gabapentin at higher dosages. Due to these properties pregabalin is seen as having higher abuse potential than gabapentin. Abuse of pregabalin is described at doses up to 20 times maximum therapeutic doses and is usually taken orally but may be taken intravenously, rectally or by smoking. The risk of gabapentinoid abuse appears to be greatest in those with a history of addiction, so caution should be exercised when prescribed in this group. The benefits of gabapentinoids are mainly in the treatment of neuropathic pain. Their use has increased largely due to off-licence use, in spite of a lack of evidence for benefit in nociceptive pain, post-operative pain, sciatica and migraine. Their benefits in neuropathic pain are modest, with most studies showing a number needed to treat of 6 to 8 to achieve a measured 50% improvement in pain.[234,235,236,237,238,239]

92. Answer a

Clostridium difficile, a gram positive, anaerobic, spore-forming, toxin producing bacillus, was officially renamed Clostridioides difficile in 2016, to reflect differences between this species and other members of the clostridium genus. It has been known as a gut commensal for many years, and its association with diarrhoeal infection has increased since the introduction of antibiotics.

Clostridioides difficile infection (CDI) is the most common cause of nosocomial diarrhoea. Those in residential care and those hospitalised are at increased risk although community infection is becoming more common. Those in acute hospitals are at greater risk than the residential care population. The theory that gastric acid suppression may increase the risk of CDI has not been proven and it has been observed that gastric acid does not kill C difficile spores. CDI most commonly occurs due to spore transmission. Spores are resistant to heat, acid and antibiotics and may survive in the environment for several months. Approximately 5% of adults and 15-70% of children are colonised by C difficile.[244]

93. Answer c

Alzheimer's disease is the most common form of dementia in those over the age of 65 years. It usually presents with a typical anterograde amnesia. Those affected often have one other cognitive domain affected, and atypical forms can present with predominantly visuospatial, language or executive features.

Although not routinely used, biomarkers can be useful in diagnosis. The underlying pathology of Alzheimer's disease of intraneuronal hyperphosphorylated tau tangles and extraneuronal amyloid β plaques can be used to aid diagnosis. A negative amyloid PET scan strongly suggests another diagnosis, although a positive test in the elderly can be more difficult to interpret with some overlap with normal variants and other pathologies. Cerebrospinal fluid may show a decrease in amyloid β and an increase in total and phosphorylated tau protein.

The first step after diagnosis is to assess patient safety and caregiver resources.[247]

94. Answer e

Direct oral anticoagulants (DOACs) are <u>more</u> effective than warfarin at reducing stroke in those with atrial fibrillation. All cause mortality is <u>decreased</u> in those on DOACs versus warfarin in those with atrial fibrillation. DOACs have a <u>lower</u> risk of major bleeding than warfarin. DOACs have a <u>lower</u> risk of intracranial bleeding than warfarin.

The risk of gastrointestinal bleeding is higher with some DOACs (dabigatran, rivaroxaban, edoxaban) than with warfarin.[248]

95. Answer d

Nikolsky's sign is elicited by applying tangential pressure with a finger or thumb to affected, peri-lesional or normal skin. It is positive if there is extension of blistering or removal of skin in the rubbed area. It reflects underlying acantholysis, which occurs when there is loss of coherence between epidermal cells due to the breakdown if intercellular bridges. It occurs in pemphigus and not pemphigoid and can be useful to differentiate the two.[252]

96. Answer c

Familial hypercholesterolaemia is a common inherited condition resulting in prolonged exposure to high LDL levels and premature cardiovascular disease. Incidence rates vary from 1 in 500 to 1 in 100 in some high-risk populations such as Ashkenazi Jews, French Canadians, Lebanese and some South African populations. In its most common form it is a monogenic autosomal dominant disorder affecting LDL receptors and therefor LDL uptake from the peripheral circulation. Typical genet c mutations will not always be found and genetic analysis and their absence should not exclude the diagnosis or delay treatment. Homozygotes may be affected as early as the first decade of life and statin treatment should be considered in all affected children, including heterozygotes. Cardiovascular risk scores underestimate risk in those with familial hypercholesterolaemia.[258]

97. Answer d

Pulmonary fibrosis has many potential causes, the most common being idiopathic pulmonary fibrosis, sarcoidosis and connective tissue associated interstitial lung disease. Idiopathic pulmonary fibrosis invariably progresses to respiratory failure and death. Over half of cases of pulmonary fibrosis from other causes will have a stable chronic disease and may improve with treatment. No standard measure for disease progression exists with varying methods used. Serological testing is not useful to assess disease progression, with other methods such as FVC measurement often used. Supplemental oxygen may be necessary in hypoxic patients. Pulmonary rehabilitation has been shown to improve symptoms and quality of life in pulmonary fibrosis. Immunosuppressive treatments may be useful in inflammation-driven disease but not in idiopathic pulmonary fibrosis.[260]

98. Answer c

Guillain Barre syndrome is a progressive motor weakness, usually symmetrical and beginning in the legs, and reaching its maximum weakness within four weeks of onset. It is assumed to be due to an immunological response to triggers such as surgery or infection. 3% of those affected will die and 25% will require mechanical ventilation. Corticosteroids are of no benefit and should not be used. Plasma exchange and intravenous immunoglobulin have become valuable disease modifying treatments due to proven benefit.

Neurological involvement and polyneuropathy were described after the previous SARS CoV1 ad MERS epidemics and also after SARS CoV2 infection, with several case reports describing post COVID-19 Guillane Barre syndrome.[267,268]

99. Answer e

Latent tuberculosis is associated with a positive tuberculin skin test and a positive interferon-γ-release assay (IGRA) test. The highest risk for transformation is in the first two years after initial infection. It is not contagious.

Risk of progression to active TB is 20 times higher in those with HIV than for the HIV-negative population.[281,282,283]

100. Answer d

The most commonly affected joints in acute gout are the 1st metatarsophalangeal joints, knees, ankles and midfoot.[288]

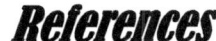

References

1. Ananthan K, Onida S, Davies AH. Nutcracker Syndrome: An Update on Current Diagnostic Criteria and Management Guidelines. Eur J Vasc Endovasc Surg. 2017 Jun;53(6):886-894.

2. Athithan L, Gulsin GS, McCann GP, Levelt E. Diabetic cardiomyopathy: Pathophysiology, theories and evidence to date. World J Diabetes. 2019 Oct 15;10(10):490-510.

3. Mikolasch TA, Garthwaite HS, Porter JC. Update in diagnosis and management of interstitial lung disease. Clin Med (Lond). 2017 Apr;17(2):146-153.

4. Thanabalasingham G, Owen KR. Diagnosis and management of maturity onset diabetes of the young (MODY). BMJ. 2011 Oct 19;343:d6044.

5. Shah SY, Higgins A, Desai MY. Bicuspid aortic valve: Basics and beyond. Cleve Clin J Med. 2018 Oct;85(10):779-784.

6. Clayton B, Morgan-Hughes G, Roobottom C. Transcatheter aortic valve insertion (TAVI): a review. Br J Radiol. 2014 Jan;87 (1033):20130595.

7. Neylon A, Ahmed K, Mercanti F, Sharif F, Mylotte D. Transcatheter aortic valve implantation: status update. J Thorac Dis. 2018 Nov;10(Suppl 30):S3637-S3645.

8. Chaturvedi S, McCrae KR Diagnosis and management of the antiphospholipid syndrome. Blood Rev. 2017 Nov;31(6):406-417.

9. Shipton MJ, Thachil J. Vitamin B12 deficiency - A 21st century perspective. Clin Med (Lond). 2015 Apr;15(2):145-50.

10. INSIGHT START Study Group, Lundgren JD, Babiker AG, Gordin F, Emery S, Grund B, Sharma S, Avihingsanon A, Cooper DA, Fätkenheuer G, Llibre JM, Molina JM, Munderi P, Schechter M, Wood R, Klingman KL, Collins S, Lane HC, Phillips AN, Neaton JD. Initiation of Antiretroviral Therapy in Early Asymptomatic HIV Infection. N Engl J Med. 2015 Aug 27;373(9):795-807.

11. Mansour D, MacPherson S. Management of decompensated cirrhosis. Clin Med (Lond) 2018 Apr 1; 18(Suppl 2) s60-65.

12. Bhatti A, Oakeshott P, Dhinoja M, Grapsa J. Ablation therapy in atrial fibrillation. BMJ. 2019 Nov 29;367:l6428.

13. Fox H, Millington L, Mahabeer I, Van Ruiten H. Duchenne muscular dystrophy. BMJ 2020;368:l7012.

14. Watson J, Mounce L, Bailey SER, Cooper SL, Hamilton W. Blood markers for cancer. BMJ 2019;367:l5774.

15. Sveren E, Agreus L, Dunn JM, Lagergren J. Peptic ulcer disease. BMJ 2019;367:l5495.

16. Kanani A, Betschel SD, Warrington R. Urticaria and angioedema. Allergy Asthma Clin Immunol. 2018 Sep 12;14(Suppl 2):59.

17. Malkud S. Telogen Effluvium: A Review. J Clin Diagn Res. 2015 Sep;9(9):WE01-3

18. Spivak JL. Myeloproliferative neoplasms. N Engl J Med 2017;376:2168-81.

19. Grigg C, Anderson D, Earnshaw J. Diagnosis and Treatment of Hereditary Hemorrhagic Telangiectasia. Ochsner J. 2017 Summer;17(2):157-161.

20. Ting DSJ, Ghosh N, Ghosh S. Herpes zoster ophthalmicus. BMJ 2019 Jan 17;364:k5234.

21. Talapko J, Škrlec I, Alebić T, Jukić M, Včev A. Malaria: The Past and the Present. Microorganisms. 2019 Jun 21;7(6).

22. Buck E, Finnigan NA. Malaria. StatPearls [Internet]. Treasure Island (FL): StatPearls Publishing; 2019 Dec 2.

23. Wilkinson IB, Raine T, Wiles K, Goodhart A, Hall C, O'Neill H. Oxford Handbook of Clinical Medicine Tenth Edition 2017. ISBN 978-0-19-968990-3.

24. Stoller JK, Lacbawan FL, Aboussouan LS. Alpha-1 Antitrypsin Deficiency. GenePeviews® [Internet]. Seattle (WA): University of Washington, Seattle; 1993-2020. 2006 Oct 27 [updated 2017 Jan 19].

25. Bird TD. Hereditary Neuropathy with Liability to Pressure Palsies. GeneReviews® [Internet]. Seattle (WA): University of Washington, Seattle; 1993-2020.1998 Sep 28 [updated 2014 Sep 25].

26. Allen KJ, Leslie SW. Autonomic Dysreflexia. StatPearls [Internet]. Treasure Island (FL): StatPearls Publishing; 2020-.2019 Jul 22.

27. Koo HK, Lawrence KA, Musini VM. Beta-blockers for preventing aortic dissection in Marfan syndrome. Cochrane Database Syst Rev. 2017 Nov 7;11:CD011103.

28. Salik I, Rawla P. Marfan Syndrome. StatPearls [Internet]. Treasure Island (FL): StatPearls Publishing; 2020 Jan-. 2019 Dec 1.

29. Allen CE, Merad M, McClain KL. Langerhans-Cell Histiocytosis. N Engl J Med. 2018 Aug 30;379(9):856-868.

30. Johns DP, Pierce R. SPIROMETRY The Measurement and Interpretation of Ventilatory Function in Clinical Practice. The Thoracic Society of Australia and New Zealand

31. Khouri J, Samaras C, Valent J, Mejia Garcia A, Faiman B, Mathur S, Hamilton K, Nakashima M, Kalaycio M. Monoclonal gammopathy of undetermined significance: A primary care guide. Cleve Clin J Med. 2019 Jan;86(1):39-46.

32. Tang Z, Chen Z, Tang B, Jiang H Primary erythromelalgia: a review. Orphanet J Rare Dis. 2015 Sep 30;10:127.

33. Schaefer TJ, Panda PK, Wolford RW. Dengue Fever. StatPearls [Internet]. Treasure Island (FL): StatPearls Publishing; 2020 -.2019 Dec 12.

34. Temprano KK. A Review of Raynaud's Disease. Mo Med. 2016 Mar-Apr;113(2):123-6.

35. https://www.who.int/news-room/fact-sheets/detail/trachoma

36. http://www.emro.who.int/health-topics/cataract/

37. Planès S, Villier C, Mallaret M. The nocebo effect of drugs. Pharmacol Res Perspect. 2016 Mar 17;4(2):e00208.

38. Alonso R, Cuevas A, Cafferata A. Diagnosis and Management of Statin Intolerance. J Atheroscler Thromb. 2019 Mar 1;26 (3):207-215.

39. Brady MF, Sundareshan V. Legionnaires' Disease (Legionella Infection). StatPearls [Internet]. Treasure Island (FL): StatPearls Publishing; 2020-.2019 Dec 30.

40. Naehrig S, Chao CM, Naehrlich L. Cystic Fibrosis. Dtsch Arztebl Int. 2017 Aug 21;114(33-34):564-574

41. Basu J, Malhotra A, Papadakis M. Exercise and hypertrophic cardiomyopathy: Two incompatible entities? Clin Cardiol. 2020;1–8

42. Cirino AL, Ho C. Hypertrophic Cardiomyopathy Overview. GeneReviews® [Internet]. Seattle (WA): University of Washington, Seattle; 1993-2020.

43. Hypertrophic Obstructive Cardiomyopathy. Dtsch Arztebl Int. 2019 Jan 25;116(4):47-53

44. Young L, Smedira NG, Tower-Rader A, Lever H, Desai MY. Hypertrophic cardiomyopathy: A complex disease. Cleve Clin J Med. 2018 May;85(5):399-411.

45. Proft F, Poddubnyy D. Ankylosing spondylitis and axial spondyloarthritis: recent insights and impact of new classification criteria. Ther Adv Musculoskelet Dis. 2018 Jun; 10(5-6): 129–139.

46. McAllister K , Goodson N , Warburton, L, Rogers G. Spondyloarthritis: diagnosis and management: summary of NICE guidance. BMJ 2017;356:j839

47. Marmor, MF, Kellner U, Lai, TYY, Melles RB, Mieler, WF. Recommendations on Screening for Chloroquine and Hydroxychloroquine Retinopathy (2016 Revision). American Academy of Ophthalmology Statement

48. Piel FB, Steinberg MH, Rees DC. Sickle Cell Disease. N Engl J Med. 2017 Apr 20;376(16):1561-1573.

49. https://www.who.int/genomics/public/geneticdiseases/en/index2.html

50. Samperi I, Lithgow K, Karavitaki N. Hyperprolactinaemia. J Clin Med. 2019 Dec 13;8(12). pii: E2203.

51. Onimoe G, Rotz S. Sickle cell disease: A primary care update. Cleve Clin J Med. 2020 Jan;87(1):19-27.

52. Jinna S, Khandhar PB. Hydroxyurea Toxicity. StatPearls [Internet]. Treasure Island (FL): StatPearls Publishing; 2020-.2019 Nov 15.

53. Agrawal R, Moghtader S, Ayyala U[1,2], Bandi V, Sharafkhaneh A. Update on management of stable chronic obstructive pulmonary disease. J Thorac Dis. 2019 Sep;11(Suppl 14):S1800-S1809.

54. Lee A, Xie YL, Barry CE, Chen RY. Current and future treatments for tuberculosis. BMJ 2020;368:m216

55, https://www.hse.ie/eng/health/immunisation/hcpinfo/guidelines/

56. Brunner-La Rocca HP, Sanders-van Wijk S. Natriuretic Peptides in Chronic Heart Failure. Card Fail Rev. 2019 Feb;5(1):44-49.

57. Taylor KS, Verbakel JY, Feakins BG, Price CP, Perera R, Bankhead C, Plüddemann A. Diagnostic accuracy of point-of-care natriuretic peptide testing for chronic heart failure in ambulatory care: systematic review and meta-analysis. BMJ. 2018 May 21;361:k1450

58. McLellan J, Heneghan CJ, Perera R, Clements AM, Glasziou PP, Kearley KE, Pidduck N, Roberts NW, Tyndel S, Wright FL, Bankhead C. B-type natriuretic peptide-guided treatment for heart failure. Cochrane Database Syst Rev. 2016 Dec;12:CD008966.

59. Penfold RS, Prendecki M, McAdoo S, Tam FW. Primary IgA nephropathy: current challenges and future prospects. Int J Nephrol Renovasc Dis. 2018 Apr 12;11:137-148.

60. Selvaskandan H, Cheung CK, Muto M, Barratt J. New strategies and perspectives on managing IgA nephropathy. Clin Exp Nephrol. 2019 May;23(5):577-588

61. Ungprasert P, Ryu JH, Matteson EL. Clinical Manifestations, Diagnosis, and Treatment of Sarcoidosis. Mayo Clin Proc Innov Qual Outcomes. 2019 Aug 2;3(3):358-375.

62. Stockton D, Doherty VR, Brewster DH. Risk of cancer in patients with dermatomyositis or polymyositis, and follow-up implications: a Scottish population-based cohort study. Br J Cancer. 2001 Jul 6;85(1):41-5.

63. Cheeti A, Panginikkod S. Dermatomyositis And Polymyositis. StatPearls [Internet]. Treasure Island (FL): StatPearls Publishing; 2020-.2019 Nov 13.

64. Farmakidis C, Pasnoor M, Dimachkie MM, Barohn RJ. Treatment of Myasthenia Gravis. Neurol Clin. 2018 May;36(2):311-337

65. Jordan A, Freimer M. Recent advances in understanding and managing myasthenia gravis. F1000Res. 2018 Oct 31;7.

66. Wang XY, Zhang F, Zhang C, Zheng LR, Yang J.The Biomarkers for Acute Myocardial Infarction and Heart Failure. Biomed Res Int. 2020 Jan 17;2020:2018035.

67. Long B, Koyfman A, Gottlieb M. Diagnosis of Acute Heart Failure in the Emergency Department: An Evidence-Based Review. West J Emerg Med. 2019 Oct 24;20(6):875-884.

68. Yin Y, Wunderink RG. MERS, SARS and other coronaviruses as causes of pneumonia. Respirology. 2018 Feb;23(2):130-137.

69. Tudor ME, Al Aboud AM, Gossman WG. Syphilis. StatPearls [Internet]. Treasure Island (FL): StatPearls Publishing; 2020-.2019 Oct 29.

70. Ghanem KG., Ram S, Rice P. The Modern Epidemic of Syphilis. N Engl J Med 2020;382:845-54.

71. Okabayashi T, Shima Y, Sumiyoshi T, Kozuki A, Ito S, Ogawa Y, Kobayashi M, Hanazaki K. Diagnosis and management of insulinoma. World J Gastroenterol. 2013 Feb 14;19(6):829-37

72. Zhuo F, Anastasopoulou C. Insulinoma. StatPearls [Internet]. Treasure Island (FL): StatPearls Publishing; 2020-.2019 Sep 3.

73. Barthel A, Benker G, Berens K, Diederich S, Manfras B, Gruber M, Kanczkowski W, Kline G, Kamvissi-Lorenz V, Hahner S, Beuschlein F, Brennand A, Boehm BO, Torpy DJ, Bornstein SR. An Update on Addison's Disease. Exp Clin Endocrinol Diabetes. 2019 Feb;127(2-03):165-175.

74. Elshimy G, Alghoula F, Jeong JM. Adrenal Crisis. StatPearls [Internet]. Treasure Island (FL): StatPearls Publishing; 2020-.2019 Aug 22

75. Rushworth RL, Torpy DJ, Falhammar H. Adrenal Crisis. N Engl J Med. 2019 Aug 29;381(9):852-861.

76. Loverdos K, Fotiadis A, Kontogianni C, Iliopoulou M, Gaga M. Lung nodules: A comprehensive review on current approach and management. Ann Thorac Med. 2019 Oct-Dec;14(4):226-238.

77. El Sabbagh A, Reddy YNV, Nishimura RA. Mitral Valve Regurgitation in the Contemporary Era: Insights Into Diagnosis, Management, and Future Directions. JACC Cardiovasc Imaging. 2018 Apr;11(4):628-643.

78. Drysdale SB, Kelly DF. How to use…respiratory viral studies. Arch Dis Child Educ Pract Ed. 2019 Oct;104(5):274-278.

79. Christin Peteranderl, PhD1 Susanne Herold, MD, PhD1 Carole Schmoldt, PhD. Human Influenza Virus Infections. Semin Respir Crit Care Med 2016;37:487–500

80. Wallace ZS, Miloslavsky EM. Management of ANCA associated vasculitis. BMJ 2020;369:m421

81. Mohandas P, Lowden M, Varma S. Bowen's disease. BMJ 2020;368:m813

82. Matthay MA, Zemans RL, Zimmerman GA, Arabi YM, Beitler JR, Mercat A, Herridge M, Randolph AG, Calfee CS. Acute respiratory distress syndrome. Nat Rev Dis Primers. 2019 Mar 14;5(1):18.

83. Mehta PA, Tolar J. Adam MP, Ardinger HH, Pagon RA, Wallace SE, Bean LJH, Stephens K, Amemiya A. Fanconi Anemia. GeneReviews® [Internet]. Seattle (WA): University of Washington, Seattle; 1993-2020. 2002 Feb 14 [updated 2018 Mar 8].

84. Young NS.. Aplastic anemia. N Engl J Med . 2018 October 25; 379(17): 1643–1656

85. Kaseb H, Hozayen S. Chromosome Instability Syndromes. StatPearls [Internet]. Treasure Island (FL): StatPearls Publishing; 2020-.2019 Aug 4

86. Savage SA. Dyskeratosis congenita. GeneReviews® [Internet]. Seattle (WA): University of Washington, Seattle; 1993-2020.

87. Clinton C, Gazda HT. Diamond-Blackfan Anemia. GeneReviews® [Internet]. Seattle (WA): University of Washington, Seattle; 1993-2020.

88. Patacsil SJ, Noor M, Leyva A. A Review of Benign Hepatic Tumors and Their Imaging Characteristics. Cureus. 2020 Jan 29;12(1):e6813.

89. Garcia HH, Nash TE, Del Brutto OH. Clinical symptoms, diagnosis, and treatment of neurocysticercosis. Lancet Neurol. 2014 Dec;13(12):1202-15.

90. Schwenkenbecher P, Wurster U, Konen FF, Gingele S, Sühs KW, Wattjes MP, Stange M, Skripuletz T. Impact of the McDonald Criteria 2017 on Early Diagnosis of Relapsing-Remitting Multiple Sclerosis. Front Neurol. 2019 Mar 15;10:188.

91. Thompson AJ, Banwell BL, Barkhof F, Carroll WM, Coetzee T, Comi G, Correale J, Fazekas F, Filippi M, Freedman MS, Fujihara K, Galetta SL, Hartung HP, Kappos L, Lublin FD, Marrie RA, Miller AE, Miller DH, Montalban X, Mowry EM, Sorensen PS, Tintoré M, Traboulsee AL, Trojano M, Uitdehaag BMJ, Vukusic S, Waubant E, Weinshenker BG, Reingold SC, Cohen JA. Diagnosis of multiple sclerosis: 2017 revisions of the McDonald criteria. Lancet Neurol. 2018 Feb;17(2):162-173.

92. Schneider JA, Cohen PR. Stevens-Johnson Syndrome and Toxic Epidermal Necrolysis: A Concise Review with a Comprehensive Summary of Therapeutic Interventions Emphasizing Supportive Measures. Adv Ther. 2017 Jun;34(6):1235-1244.

93. Parente L. Deflazacort: therapeutic index, relative potency and equivalent doses versus other corticosteroids. BMC Pharmacol Toxicol. 2017 Jan 5;18(1):1.

94. Hui DSC, Zumla A. Severe Acute Respiratory Syndrome: Historical, Epidemiologic, and Clinical Features. Infect Dis Clin North Am. 2019 Dec;33(4):869-889.

95. Chaudhry SB, Veve MP, Wagner JL. Cephalosporins: A Focus on Side Chains and β-Lactam Cross-Reactivity. Pharmacy (Basel). 2019 Jul 29;7(3). pii: E103.

96. Devchand M, Jason A Trubiano. Penicillin allergy: a practical approach to assessment and prescribing. Aust Prescr. 2019 Dec;42(6):192-199.

97. Isaacs M, Cardones AR, Rahnama-Moghadam S. DRESS syndrome: clinical myths and pearls. Cutis. 2018 Nov;102(5):322-326.

98. Bedoui Y, Guillot X, Sélambarom J, Guiraud P, Giry C, Jaffar-Bandjee MC, Ralandison S, Gasque P. Methotrexate an Old Drug with New Tricks. Int J Mol Sci. 2019 Oct 10;20(20).

99. Knowles MR, Zariwala M, Leigh M. Primary Ciliary Dyskinesia. Clin Chest Med. 2016 Sep;37(3):449-61.

100. Sharma G, Carter YM. Pectus Excavatum. StatPearls [Internet]. Treasure Island (FL): StatPearls Publishing; 2020 Jan-.2020 Jan 21.

101. Brochhausen C, Turial S, Müller FK, Schmitt VH, Coerdt W, Wihlm JM, Schier F, Kirkpatrick CJ. Pectus excavatum: history, hypotheses and treatment options. Interact Cardiovasc Thorac Surg. 2012 Jun;14(6):801-6.

102. Oladiran O, Nwosu I. Stroke risk stratification in atrial fibrillation: a review of common risk factors. J Community Hosp Intern Med Perspect. 2019 Apr; 9(2): 113–120.

103. Bagherani N, Smoller BR. An overview of cutaneous T cell lymphomas. F1000Res 2016 Jul 28;5. pii: F1000 Faculty Rev-1882.

104. Cook Shukla L, Schulze J, Farlow J, Pankratz ND, Wojcieszek J, Foroud T. Parkinson Disease Overview. GeneReviews® [Internet]. Seattle (WA): University of Washington, Seattle; 1993-2020. 2004 May 25 [updated 2019 Jul 25]

105. Caio G, Volta U, Sapone A, Leffler DA, De Giorgio R, Catassi C, Fasano A. Celiac disease: a comprehensive current review. BMC Med. 2019 Jul 23;17(1):142

106. Kolb L, Barazi H, Rosario-Collazo JA. Lipoma. StatPearls [Internet]. Treasure Island (FL): StatPearls Publishing; 2020-.2020 Jan 13.

107. Byrne CD, Patel ,J Scorletti E, Targher G. Tests for diagnosing and monitoring non-alcoholic fatty liver disease in adults. BMJ 2018;362:k2734.

108. Parthasarathy G, Revelo X, Malhi H. Pathogenesis of Nonalcoholic Steatohepatitis: An Overview. Hepatol Commun. 2020 Jan 14;4(4):478-492.

109. Shlomo Melmed, M.D. Pituitary-Tumor Endocrinopathies. N Engl J Med 2020;382:937-50.

110. Kong EL, Fowler JB. Rinne Test. StatPearls [Internet]. Treasure Island (FL): StatPearls Publishing; 2020-.2019 Jun 1.

111. Wahid NWB, Attia M. Weber Test. StatPearls [Internet]. Treasure Island (FL): StatPearls Publishing; 2020 Jan-.2020 Feb 14.

112. Chaudhry HS, Singh G. Cushing Syndrome. StatPearls [Internet]. Treasure Island (FL): StatPearls Publishing; 2020-.2019 Dec 14.

113. Newbronner E, Atkin K. The changing health of Thalidomide survivors as they age: A scoping review. Disabil Health J. 2018 Apr;11(2):184-191.

114. Cross AR, Baldwin VM, Roy S, Essex-Lopresti AE, Prior JL, Harmer NJ. Zoonoses under our noses. Microbes Infect. 2019 Jan - Feb;21(1):10-19.

115. Rodriguez-Castro KI, Franceschi M, Noto A, Miraglia C, Nouvenne A, Leandro G, Meschi T, De' Angelis GL, Di Mario F. Clinical manifestations of chronic atrophic gastritis. Acta Biomed. 2018 Dec 17;89(8-S):88-92

116. Lahner E, Carabotti M, Annibale B. Treatment of Helicobacter pylori infection in atrophic gastritis. World J Gastroenterol. 2018 Jun 14;24(22):2373-2380.

117. Minalyan A, Benhammou JN, Artashesyan A, Lewis MS, Pisegna JR. Autoimmune atrophic gastritis: current perspectives. Clin Exp Gastroenterol. 2017 Feb 7;10:19-27

118. List of Classifications – IARC Monographs

119. Constantinou CA, Fragoulis GE, Nikiphorou E. Hidradenitis suppurativa: infection, autoimmunity, or both? Ther Adv Musculoskelet Dis. 2019 Dec 30;11:1759720X19895488.

120. Drago F, Ciccarese G, Rebora A, Broccolo F, Parodi A. Pityriasis Rosea: A Comprehensive Classification. Dermatology. 2016;232(4):431-7.

121. Jefferson T, Jones MA, Doshi P, Del Mar CB, Hama R, Thompson MJ, Spencer EA, Onakpoya I. Neuraminidase inhibitors for preventing and treating influenza in healthy adults and children. Cochrane Database Syst Rev. 2014 Apr 10;(4):CD008965

122. Insogna KL. Primary Hyperparathyroidism. N Engl J Med. 2018 Sep 13;379(11):1050-1059.

123. Suresh Babu K, Kastelik J, Morjaria JB. Role of long term antibiotics in chronic respiratory diseases. Respir Med. 2013 Jun;107(6):800-15.

124. Echt DS, Ruskin JN. Use of Flecainide for the Treatment of Atrial Fibrillation. Am J Cardiol. 2020 Apr 1;125(7):1123-1133

125. Gandhi RT, Lynch JB, Del Rio C.. Mild or Moderate Covid-19. N Engl J Med. 2020 Apr 24.

126. Saadoun D, Wechsler B. Behçet's disease. Orphanet J Rare Dis. 2012 Apr 12;7:20.

127. Michos ED, McEvoy JW, Blumenthal RS. Lipid Management for the Prevention of Atherosclerotic Cardiovascular Disease. N Engl J Med. 2019 Oct 17;381(16):1557-1567.

128. Pericleous M, Kelly C. The clinical management of hereditary haemochromatosis. Frontline Gastroenterol. 2018 Apr;9(2):110-114

129. Shanbhag S, Ambinder RF. Hodgkin lymphoma: A review and update on recent progress. CA Cancer J Clin. 2018 Mar;68(2):116-132

130. Sureda A, Martínez C. Classical Hodgkin's Lymphoma. The EBMT Handbook: Hematopoietic Stem Cell Transplantation and Cellular Therapies [Internet]. 7th edition. Cham (CH): Springer; 2019. Chapter 88

131. Veauthier B, Hornecker JR. Crohn's Disease: Diagnosis and Management. Am Fam Physician. 2018 Dec 1;98(11):661-669.

132. Bonsignore M. Sleep apnea and its role in transportation safety. F1000 Research 2017, 6(F1000 Faculty Rev):2168.

133. Schiza SE, Bouloukaki I. Screening for obstructive sleep apnoea in professional drivers. Breathe (Sheff). 2020 Mar;16(1):29364

134. Razvi S, Jabbar A, Pingitore A, Danzi S, Biondi B, Klein I, Peeters R, Zaman A, Iervasi G. Thyroid Hormones and Cardiovascular Function and Diseases. J Amer Coll Cardiol. 2018 Apr 24;71(16):1781-1796.

135. Weitz JI, Fredenburgh JC, Eikelboom JW. A Test in Context: D-Dimer. J Am Coll Cardiol. 2017 Nov 7;70(19):2411-2420.

136. Bartholomew JR. Update on the management of venous thromboembolism. Cleve Clin J Med. 2017 Dec;84(12 Suppl 3):39-46.

137. Zabalza Estévez RJ, Unanue López F. Harlequin syndrome, a rare neurological disease. Neurologia. 2015 Apr;30(3):185-7

138. Feldmann H, Sprecher A, Geisbert TW. Ebola. N Engl J Med 2020;382:1832-42

139. Davidson A, Raviendran N, Murali CN, Myint PK. Managing heart failure with preserved ejection fraction. Ann Transl Med. 2020 Mar;8(6):395.

140. Diab J, Bannan A, Pollitt T. Necrotising fasciitis. BMJ 2020;369:m1428

141. El-Qushayri AE, Khalaf KM, Dahy A, Mahmoud AR, Benmelouka AY, Ghozy S, Mahmoud MU, Bin-Jumah M, Alkahtani S, Abdel-Daim MM. Fournier's gangrene mortality: A 17-year systematic review and meta-analysis. Int J Infect Dis. 2020 Mar;92:218-225

142. Ungaro R, Mehandru S, Allen PB, Peyrin-Biroulet L, Colombel JF. Ulcerative colitis. Lancet. 2017 Apr 29;389(10080):1756-1770.

143. Holland TL, Baddour LM, Bayer AS, Hoen B, Miro JM, Fowler VG Jr. Infective endocarditis. Nat Rev Dis Primers. 2016 Sep 1;2:16059

144. Cahill TJ, Baddour LM, Habib G, Hoen B, Salaun E, Pettersson GB, Schäfers HJ, Prendergast BD. Challenges in Infective Endocarditis. J Am Coll Cardiol. 2017 Jan 24;69(3):325-344

145. Yandrapalli S, Aronow WS. Cardiovascular benefits of the newer medications for treating type 2 diabetes mellitus. J Thorac Dis 2017;9(7):2124-2134

146. Piel FB, Weatherall DJ. The alpha thalassaemias. N Engl J Med 2014;371:1908-16.

147. DeFronzo R, Fleming GA, Chen K, Bicsak TA. Metformin-associated lactic acidosis: Current perspectives on causes and risk. Metabolism. 2016 Feb;65(2):20-9

148. Zeiser R, Blazar BR. Acute Graft-versus-Host Disease - Biologic Process, Prevention, and Therapy. N Engl J Med. 2017 Nov 30;377(22):2167-2179

149. Berlin DA, Gulick RM, Martinez FJ. Severe Covid-19. N Eng J Med May 15th 2020.

150. Pierre Amarenco, M.D. Transient Ischemic Attack. N Engl J Med 382;20

151. Watson J, Whiting PF, Brush JE. Interpreting a covid-19 test result. BMJ 2020;369:m1808.

152. Belay Y, Yirdaw K, Enawgaw B.. Tumor Lysis Syndrome in Patients With Hematological Malignancies. J Oncol. 2017;2017:9684909.

153. Immunisation Guidelines – National Immunisation Advisory Committee. https://www.hse.ie/eng/health/immunisation/hcpinfo/guidelines/

154. Andrew S. Bombacka Fernando C. Fervenzab. Membranous Nephropathy: Approaches to Treatment. Am J Nephrol 2018;47(suppl 1):30–42

155. Lai WL, Yeh TH, Chen PM, Chan CK, Chiang WC, Chen YM, Wu KD, Tsai TJ. Membranous Nephropathy: A Review on the Pathogenesis, Diagnosis, and Treatment. J Formos Med Assoc. 2015 Feb;114(2):102-11.Feb;114(2):102-11.

156. Riario Sforza GG, Marinou A. Hypersensitivity pneumonitis: a complex lung disease. Clin Mol Allergy. 2017 Mar 7;15:6.

157. P Spagnolo, G Rossi, A Cavazza, M Bonifazi, I Paladini, F Bonella, N Sverzellati, U Costabel. Hypersensitivity Pneumonitis: A Comprehensive Review. J Investig Allergol Clin Immunol 2015;25(4):237-50;

158. Rendon A, Schakel A. Psoriasis pathogenesis and treatment. Int J Mol Sci 2019 Mar 23;20(6):1475

159. Kimberly A. Prather, Chia C. Wang, Robert T. Schooley. Reducing transmission of SARS-CoV-2. Science 27-May-2020.

160. Khosla S, Hofbauer LC. Osteoporosis treatment: recent developments and ongoing challenges. Lancet Diabetes Endocrinol. 2027 Nov;(11):898-907

161. DiMeglio LA, Evans-Molina C, Oram RA. Type 1 diabetes. Lancet. 2018 Jun 16;391(10138):2449-2462.

162. Wilkins T, Malcolm JK, Raina D, Schade RR. Hepatitis C: diagnosis and treatment. Am Fam Physician. 2010 Jun 1;81 (11):1351-7.

163. Guss D, Sherigar J, Rosen P, Mohanty SR. Diagnosis and Management of Hepatitis C Infection in Primary Care Settings. J Gen Intern Med 33(4):551–7.

164. Wasserman A. Diagnosis and Management of Rheumatoid Arthritis. Am Fam Physician. 2011. PMID: 22150658

165. Lin YJ, Anzaghe M, Schülke S. Update on the Pathomechanism, Diagnosis, and Treatment Options for Rheumatoid Arthritis. Cells 2020 Apr 3;9(4):880.

166. Castells M, Khan DA, Phillips EJ Penicillin Allergy. N Engl J Med 2019;381:2338-51.

167. Vasanwala FF, Ong CY, Aw CWD, How CH. Management of Scabies. Singapore Med J. 2019 Jun;60(6):281-285.

168. Dressler C, Rosumeck S, Sunderkötter C, Werner RN, Nast A. The Treatment of Scabies. Dtsch Arztebl Int. 2016 Nov 14;113(45):757-762.

169. Gitlin M. Lithium Side Effects and Toxicity: Prevalence and Management Strategies. Int J Bipolar Disord. 2016 Dec;4 (1):27.

170. Orange JS. Natural Killer Cell Deficiency. J Allergy Clin Immunol. 2013 Sep;132(3):515-525.

171. Raje N, Dinakar C. Overview of Immunodeficiency Disorders. Immunol Allergy Clin North Am. 2015 Nov;35(4):599-623.

172. Catherine M Biggs, Elie Haddad, Thomas B Issekutz, Chaim M Roifman, Stuart E Turvey Newborn Screening for Severe Combined Immunodeficiency: A Primer for Clinicians. CMAJ 2017 Dec 18;189(50):E1551-E1557

173. Pathak S, McDermott MF, Savic S Autoinflammatory Diseases: Update on Classification Diagnosis and Management. J Clin Pathol. 2017 Jan;70(1):1-8.

174. R Yazdani, S Habibi, L Sharifi, G Azizi, H Abolhassani, P Olbrich, A Aghamohammadi. Common Variable Immunodeficiency: Epidemiology, Pathogenesis, Clinical Manifestations, Diagnosis, Classification, and Management. J Investig Allergol Clin Immunol 2020;30(1):14-34.

175. Bull MJ. Down Syndrome. N Engl J Med 2020;382:2344-52.

176. Roubinian N. TACO and TRALI: Biology, Risk Factors, and Prevention Strategies. Hematology Am Soc Hematol Educ Program 2018 Nov 30;2018(1):585-594.

177. Yozamp, N, Hornick, JL, Chiodo CP,Miller, AL, Loscalzo, J. The game is afoot. N Engl J Med 2020; 382:2249-2255

178. Holland J, Bernstein J. Bell Palsy. Am Fam Physician. 2011 Oct 15;84(8):947-3.

179. Rybstein MD, DeSancho, MT. Hypercoagulable States and Thrombophilias: Risks Relating to Recurrent Venous Thromboembolism. Semin Intervent Radiol 2018;35:99–104.

180. Salvagno GL, Pavan C, Lippi G. Rare thrombophilic conditions. Ann Transl Med. 2018 Sep;6(17):342

181. Ramanujam VS, Anderson KE. Porphyria Diagnostics-Part 1: A Brief Overview of the Porphyrias. Curr Protoc Hum Genet. 2015 Jul 1;86:17.20.1-17.20.26.

182. Reid IR. Recent advances in understanding and managing Paget's disease. F1000Res. 2019. PMID: 31489180

183. Nebot Valenzuela E, et al. Epidemiology and pathology of Paget's disease of bone - a review. Wien Med Wochenschr. 2017. PMID: 27600564

184. Davis BM, et al. Everything You Always Wanted to Know About Rabies Virus (But Were Afraid to Ask).. Annu Rev Virol. 2015. PMID: 26958924

185. Zhu S, Guo C. Rabies Control and Treatment: From Prophylaxis to Strategies with Curative Potential. Viruses 2016, 8, 279

186. Koury R, Warrington SJ. Rabies. StatPearls [Internet]. Treasure Island (FL): StatPearls Publishing; 2020 Jan.

187. Paropola P. Bedbugs. N Engl J Med 2020;382:2230-7.

188. De Leo S, Lee SY, Braverman LE. Hyperthyroidism. Lancet 2016 Aug 27;388(10047):906-918.

189. Qi C, Mao X, Zhang Z, Wu H. Classification and differential diagnosis of diabetic nephropathy.J Diabetes Res. 2017;2017:8637138.

190. Kopel J, Pena-Hernandez C, Nugent K. Evolving Spectrum of Diabetic Nephropathy. World J Diabetes. 2019 May 15;10 (5):269-279.

191. Fioretto P, Mauer M. HISTOPATHOLOGY OF DIABETIC NEPHROPATHY. Semin Nephrol. 2007 March ; 27(2): 195–207

192. Wrenn SM, Vaidya A,. Lubitz CC. Primary aldosteronism. Gland Surg 2020;9(1):14-24

193. Kamilaris CDC, Stratakis CA. An update on adrenal endocrinology: significant discoveries in the last 10 years and where the field is heading in the next decade. Hormones (2018) 17:479–490

194. Horby P, Lim WS, Emberson J Est al. Effect of dexamethasone in hospitalised patients with COVID 19: preliminary report. medRxiv 2020.06.22.20137273 (Preprint.) 2020.

195. Beigel JH, Tomashek MPH, Dodd LE et al. Remdesivir for the treatment of COVID 19 - preliminary report. N Engl J Med May 22 2020.

196. Cao B, Wang Y, Wen D et al. A trial of lopinavir-ritonavir in adults hospitalised with severe COVID 19. N Engl J Med 2020; 382:1787-1799.

197. Fauci AS, Lane HC. Four decades of HIV/AIDS - much accomplished, much to do. N Engl J Med 383;1.

198. Theodore N. Degenerative Cervical Spondylosis. N Engl J Med 2020;383:159-68

199. Kipps TJ, et al. Chronic lymphocytic leukaemia. Nat Rev Dis Primers 2017 Jan 19;3:16096.

200. Chronic lymphocytic leukemia: 2017 update on diagnosis, risk stratification, and treatment. Hallek M.Am J Hematol. 2017 Sep;92(9):946-965

201. Liam CK, Andarini S, Lee P, Ho JC, Chau NQ, Tscheikuna J. Lung cancer staging now and in the f uture.Respirology. 2015 May;20(4):526-34.

202. Hirsch FR, et al Lung cancer: current therapies and new targeted treatments. Lancet. 2017. PMID: 27574741 Free article. Review

203. INTERNATIONAL ASSOCIATION FOR THE STUDY OF LUNG CANCER 8th Edition of the TNM Classification for Lung Cancer. https://www.iaslc.org/Portals/0/35348-cards-erx_combined_trap_card3_1_copy.pdf?ver=2019-05-22-154420-317

204. Vorselaars VMM, Hosman AE, Westermann CJJ, Snijder RJ, Mager JJ, Goumans MJ, Post MC Pulmonary Arterial Hypertension and Hereditary Haemorrhagic Telangiectasia. Int J Mol Sci. 2018 Oct 17;19(10):3203.

205. Hoeper MM, et al Pulmonary Hypertension. Dtsch Arztebl Int. 2017.

206. Neumann V, Löseke S, Nowak D, Herth FJF, Tannapfel A. Malignant pleural mesothelioma incidence, etiology, diagnosis, treatment, and occupational health. Dtsch Arztebl Int 2013; 110(18): 319□26.

207. Deepak MW Balak Enes Hajdarbegovic. Drug-induced psoriasis: clinical perspectives. Psoriasis: Targets and Therapy 2017:7 87–94

208. Członkowska A, et al. Wilson disease. Nat Rev Dis Primers. 2018. PMID: 30190489

209. Diabetes insipidus. Levy M, Prentice M, Wass J. Diabetes insipidus BMJ 2019;364:l321

210. Filippatos TD, Makri A, Elisaf MS, Liamis G Hyponatremia in the elderly: challenges and solutions. Clin Interv Aging. 2017 Nov 14;12:1957-1965.

211. Walker A Pottinger G, Scott A, Hopkins, C. Anosmia and loss of smell during the covid-19 pandemic. BMJ 25 July-1 August 2020

212. Cleverley J, Piper J, Jones MM. The role of chest radiography in confirming Covid-19 pneumonia. BMJ 2020;370:m2426

213. Hadjieconomou S, Hughes J. Covid-19 associated chilblain-like lesions in an asymptomatic doctor. BMJ 2020;370

214. Nicholson TW, Talbot NP, Nickol A, Chadwick AJ, Lawton O. Respiratory failure and non-invasive respiratory support during the covid-19 pandemic: an update for re-deployed hospital doctors and primary care physicians. BMJ 2020;369:m2446

215. https://www.hse.ie/eng/health/immunisation/hcpinfo/guidelines/chapter22.pdf

216. Okafor CN, et al. Bacillus Calmette Guerin (BCG). StatPearls. 2020 Jan–. PMID: 30844212

217. http://www.hpra.ie/docs/default-source/default-document-library/bcg-medac-(bacillus-calmette-gu%C3%A9rin-for-intravesical-use)---important-safety-information-from-medac-gmbh-as-approved-by-the-hpra.pdf?sfvrsn=0

218. Chambers HF, Bayer AS. Native valve infective endocarditis. N Eng J Med 383;6

219. Camellino D, Dejaco C. Update on treatment of polymyalgia rheumatica. Reumatismo 2018;70(1):59-66

220. Guggino G, Ferrante A, Macaluso F, Triolo G, Ciccia F. Pathogenesis of polymyalgia rheumatica. Reumatismo 2018:70 (1):10-17

221. Dejaco C, Brouwer E, Mason JC, Buttergereit F, Mtteson EL, Dasgupta B. Giant cell arteritis and polymyalgia rheumatica – current challenges and opportunities. Nat Rev Rheumatol 2017 Oct;13(10)578-592

222. Arnold AC, Ng J, Raj SR. Postural tachycardia syndrome - Diagnosis, physiology, and prognosis. Auton Neurosci. 2018 Dec;215:3-11.

223. Syx D, et al. Hypermobility, the Ehlers-Danlos syndromes and chronic pain. Clin Exp Rheumatol. 2017. PMID: 28967365

224. Cruccu G, Di Stefano G, Truini A. Trigeminal neuralgia. N Engl J Med 2020;383:754-62.

225. Greenhalgh T,Knight M, A'Court C, Buxton M, Husain L. Management of post-acute covid-19 in primary care. BMJ 2020;370:m3026

226. Simunovic MP. Colour vision deficiency. Eye (2010) 24, 747–755

227. Dain SJ. Clinical colour vision tests. Clin Exp Optom 2004; 87: 4-5: 276293.

228. Fisher SB, et al The incidental thyroid nodule. CA Cancer J Clin. 2018;68:97-105.

229. Haugen BR, et a. 2015 American Thyroid Association Management Guidelines for Adult Patients with Thyroid Nodules and Differentiated Thyroid Cancer: The American Thyroid Association Guidelines Task Force on Thyroid Nodules and Differentiated Thyroid Cancer. THYROID Volume 26, Number 1, 2016

230. Ashcroft J, Fraser E, Krishnamoorthy S, Westwood Ruttledge S. Carbon monoxide poisoning. BMJ 2019;365:2299.

231. Purohit T, Cappell MS. Primary biliary cirrhosis: Pathophysiology, clinical presentation and therapy. World J Hepatol 2015 May 8;7(7):926-41

232. Postema PG, et al. The measurement of the QT interval. Current Cardiology Reviews, 2014, 10, 287-294

233. Crotti L, Celano G, Dagradi F, Schwartz PJ. Congenital long QT syndrome. Orphanet J Rare Dis. 2008 Jul 7;3:18.

234. Pregabalin for acute and chronic pain in adults. Moore RA, Straube S, Wiffen PJ, Derry S, McQuay HJ. Cochrane Database of Systemic Reviews. Issue 3, Art. No.: CD007076. doi: 10.1002/14651858.CD007076.pub2.

235. Pharmacotherapy for neuropathic pain in adults: a systematic review and meta analysis. Finnerup B et al. The Lancet Neurology. Vol. 14, Issue 2. 162-173. doi: 10.1016/S1474-4422(14)70251-0

236. Single dose oral gabapentin for established acute post operative pain in adults (Review). Straube S, Derry S, Moore RA, Wiffen PJ, McQuay HJ. Cochrane Database of Systemic Reviews 2010, Issue 5. Art No: CD008183

237. Gabapentin or pregabalin for the prophylaxis of episodic migraine in adults (Review). Linde M, Mulleners WM, Chronicle EP, McRory DC. Cochrane Database of Systemic Reviews 2013. Issue 6, Art No: CD010609

238. Antiepileptic drugs for neuropathic pain and fibromyalgia – an overview of Cochrane reviews (Review). Wiffen PJ, Derry S, Moore RA, Aldington D, Cole P, Rice ASC, Lunn MPT, Hamunen K, Haanpaa M, Kalso EA. Cochrane Databse of Sytematic Reviews 2013, Issue 11, Art No: CD010567

239. Misuse and Abuse of Pregabalin and Gabapentin: Cause for Concern? Schifano F. CNS Drugs (2014) 26:491-196. doi 10.1007/s40263-014-0164-4

240. AES Position Statement on Generic Substitution of Antiepileptic Drugs. Vossler DG, Anderson GD, Bainbridge J. Epilepsy Curr. 2016 May-Jun;16(3):209-11. doi: 10.5698/1535-7511-16.3.209

241. Generic substitution of antiepileptic drugs: a systematic review of prospective and retrospective studies. Yamada M, Welty TE Ann Pharmacother. 2011 Nov;45(11):1406-15. doi: 10.1345/aph.1Q349. Epub 2011 Oct 25

242. Clinical Equivalence of Generic and Brand-Name Drugs Used in Cardiovascular Disease: A Systematic Review and Meta-analysis Aaron S. Kesselheim, MD, JD, MPH, Alexander S. Misono, BA, Joy L. Lee, BA, Margaret R. Stedman, MPH, M. Alan Brookhart, PhD, Niteesh K. Choudhry, MD, PhD, and William H. Shrank, MD, MSHS. JAMA. 2008 December 3; 300(21): 2514–2526. doi:10.1001/jama.2008.758.

243. Generic versus brand-name drugs used in cardiovascular diseases.Manzoli L, Flacco ME, Boccia S, D'Andrea E, Panic N, Marzuillo C, Siliquini R, Ricciardi W, Villari P, Ioannidis JP. Eur J Epidemiol. 2016 Apr;31(4):351-68. doi: 10.1007/s10654-015-0104-8. Epub 2015 Nov 30

244. Czepiel J, et al Clostridium difficile infection: review. Eur J Clin Microbiol Infect Dis (2019) 38:1211–1221

245. Bosch FTM , Di Nisio M, Büller HR, van Es N. Diagnostic and Therapeutic Management of Upper Extremity Deep Vein Thrombosis. J. Clin. Med. 2020, 9, 2069

246. Hsu WH, et al. Insights into the management of gastric antral vascular ectasia (watermelon stomach). Therap Adv Gastroenterol. 2018 Jan 14;11:1756283X17747471

247. Ljubenkov PA, et al. Dementia. Semin Neurol 2016;36:397–404.

248. NB Medical Education Hot Topic. Atrial Fibrillation. assets/31/C31BEAAC-C835-4726-80D67923B52F27C6_document/Hot_Topic_Atrial_Fibrillation__July_2020.pdf

249. John A,Canaday DH. Herpes zoster in the older adult. Infect Dis Clin North Am. 2017 December ; 31(4): 811–826.

250. Yamagami J. Recent advances in the understanding and treatment of pemphigus and pemphigoid [version 1; referees: 2 approved] F1000Research 2018, 7(F1000 Faculty Rev):1360

251. Miyamoto D, Santi CG, Aoki V, Maruta CW. Bullous pemphigoid. An Bras Dermatol. 2019;94(2):133-46

252. Seshadri D, Kumaran M S, Kanwar AJ. Acantholysis revisited: Back to basics. Indian J Dermatol Venereol Leprol 2013;79:120-6

253. HOT TOPIC ~ STROKE AND TIA NB MEDICAL EDUCATION. assets/30/F40305A7-4543-465A-B25A0081130F6C2D_document/NB_Med_Sroke_and_TIA__Sep_2020_.pdf

254. HOT TOPIC ~ BELL'S PALSY NB MEDICAL EDUCATION. /assets/44/964F4183-8027-45BC-81CEDE9E9CCC07A8_document/NB_Med_Bell_s_Palsy__Dec_2019__21955_.pdf

255. HOT TOPIC ~ CHRONIC OBSTRUCTIVE PULMONARY DISEASE NB MEDICAL EDUCATION.assets/4/BE304FA1-55DE-40D6- 9B4B0704290CAE03_document/NB_Med_COPD__Nov_2019_.pdf

256. HOT TOPIC VENOUS THROMBOEMBOLISM NB MEDICAL EDUCATION

257. Gatselis NK, Zachou K, Koukoulis GK, Dalekos GNAutoimmune hepatitis, one disease with many faces: etiopathogenetic, clinico-laboratory and histological characteristics. World J Gastroenterol. 2015 Jan 7;21(1):60-83.

258. Bouhairie VE, Goldberg AC. Familial hypercholesterolemia. Cardiol Clin. 2015 May ; 33(2): 169–179

259. Kumar A, et al. Simple Partial Seizure. StatPearls. 2020 Jan–. PMID: 29763181

260. Wijsenbeek M, Cottin V. Spectrum of Fibrotic Lung Diseases. N Engl J Med 2020;383:958-68

261. Schmieder SJ, et al Keratosis Follicularis (Darier Disease). StatPearls. 2020 Jan–. PMID: 30137841

262. Schmieder SJ, et al Keratosis Follicularis (Darier Disease). StatPearls. 2020 Jan–. PMID: 30137841

263. Balatsouras DG, et al. Benign paroxysmal positional vertigo in the elderly: current insights. Clin Interv Aging 2018 Nov 5;13:2251-2266.

264. Hickman Pepmueller P. Undifferentiated Connective Tissue Disease, Mixed Connective Tissue Disease, and Overlap Syndromes in Rheumatology. Mo Med. Mar-Apr 2016;113(2):136-40.

265. Holdgate N, St Clair EW. Recent advances in primary Sjogren's syndrome. F1000Res. 2016 Jun 17;5:F1000 Faculty Rev-1412.

266. Rongioletti F, Ferreli C, Atzori L, Bottoni U, Soda G. Scleroderma with an update about clinico-pathological correlation. G Ital Dermatol Venereol. 2018 Apr;153(2):208-215.

267. Rahimi K. Guillain-Barre syndrome during COVID-19 pandemic: an overview of the reports. Neurol Sci 2020 Sep 2.

268. Walling AD, Dickson G. Guillain-Barré syndrome. Am Fam Physician 2013 Feb 1;87(3):191-7.

269. Ahmed M. Acute cholangitis - an update. World J Gastrointest Pathophysiol 2018 February 15; 9(1): 1-7.

270. Bergmann C, Guay-Woodford LM, Harris PC, Horie S, DJM, Torres VE. Polycystic kidney disease. Nat Rev Dis Primers; 4 (1): 50.

271. Leebeek FWG, Eikenboom JCJ. Von Willebrand's Disease. N Engl J Med 375;21

272. Mehravar M, Shirazi A, Nazari M, Banan M. Mosaicism in CRISPR/Cas9-mediated genome editing. Developmental Biology 445 (2019) 156-162.

273. Butler AE, Misselbrook D. Distinguishing between type 1 and type 2 diabetes. s: BMJ 2020;370:m2998

274. Nigwekar SU, Thadhani R, Brandenburg VM. Calciphylaxis. N Engl J Med 2018;378:1704-14

275. Zhong J Yang HC, Fogo AB. A perspective on chronic kidney disease progression. Am J Physiol Renal Physiol. 2017 Mar 1;312(3):F375-F384.

276. Chawla LS, Eggers PW, Ph.D., Star RA Kimmel PL Acute Kidney Injury and Chronic Kidney Disease as Interconnected Syndromes. N Engl J Med 2014;371:58-66.

277. HOW TO DO IT Skin prick testing. Occupational Medicine 2019;69:298–299.

278. Nemakayala DR; Ramphul K. Caplan syndrome. StatPearls Publishing; 2019 Mar 14.

279. Stephens DS, McElrath MJ. COVID-19 and the Path to Immunity. JAMA. Published online September 11, 2020

280. Tyler KL. Acute Viral Encephalitis. N Engl J Med 379;6

281. Pai M, Alice Zwerling A, Menzies D,. Systematic Review: T-Cell–based Assays for the Diagnosis of Latent Tuberculosis Infection: An Update. Ann Intern Med. 2008 August 05; 149(3): 177–184

282. Bastian I, Coulter C and the National Tuberculosis Advisory Committee (NTAC)Position statement on interferon-γ release assays for the detection of latent tuberculosis infection.

283. Suárez I, Fünger SM, Kröger S, Rademacher J, Fätkenheuer G, Rybniker J. The Diagnosis and Treatment of Tuberculosis. Dtsch Arztebl Int 2019; 116: 729–35

284. Petersen LR, Brault AC, Nasci RS. West Nile Virus: Review of the Literature Lyle R. Petersen, MD, MPH, Aaron C. Brault, PhD, and Roger S. Nasci, PhD. JAMA. 2013 July 17; 310(3): 308–315.

285. Ulbert S. West Nile virus vaccines – current situation and future directions. HUMAN VACCINES & IMMUNOTHERAPEUTICS 2019, VOL. 15, NO. 10, 2337–2342

286. Horvatits T, Schulze zur Wiesch J, Lütgehetmann M, Lohse AW, Pischke S. The Clinical Perspective on Hepatitis E. Viruses 2019, 11, 617;

287. Simonetto DA, Gines P, Kamath PS. Hepatorenal syndrome: pathophysiology, diagnosis, and management

288. Abhishek A, Roddy E, Doherty M. Gout - a guide for the general and acute physicians. Clin Med (Lond) 2017 Feb;17(1):54-59

289. Merwick A, Werring D. Posterior circulation ischaemic stroke. BMJ 2014; 348: g3175

290. Ortiz A et al. Fabry disease revisited: Management and treatment recommendations for adult patients. Molecular Genetics and Metabolism 123 (2018) 416–427417

291. Christopher Nicholas Floyd1,2Time to review fibrate prescribing? Drug and Therapeutics Bulletin | October 2019 | VOL 57 | NO 10

292. Reboli AC, Farrar WE. Erysipelothrix rhusiopathiae: an occupational pathogen. Clin Microbiol Rev. 1989 Oct;2(4):354-9

293. Page CP, Fitzgerald B, Hawes EM. Latent autoimmune diabetes of adulthood: case report. Clin Diabetes Endocrinol. 2017 Nov 28;3:11.

294. Devarbhav H. An Update on Drug-induced Liver Injury. Journal of Clinical and Experimental Hepatology | September 2012 | Vol. 2 | No. 3 | 247–259.

295. Vu DM, et al Chikungunya Virus. Clin Lab Med 37 (2017) 371–382